Early Detection, Better Outcomes: New Tool Enhances Breast Cancer Conservative Treatment

Namita

First Printing, 2024

Contents

Chapter 1

Introduction

This chapter introduces the context, motivation and objectives behind this project book. We created an outline to describe the main contents of each chapter.

1.1 Context

Breast cancer is one of the most common diseases in the world and is characterised by the fast evolution that normally occurs. In the last years, we have been watching great progress in the way this disease is treated and planned. A reason for that is the existence of breast cancer routines screening habits that permit that most of the cancers detected at an early stage can be treated with great efficacy by conservatives approaches, most known as (Breast Cancer Conservative Treatment (BCCT)). The BCCT approach to breast cancer is developing very efficiently. Almost every breast cancer (near 90%) that has an early diagnosis can be treated and cured successfully [81, 82, 101]. This treatment is focused on the aesthetic results of the surgery and on improving the quality of life of people who suffered from this disease. In the past, this assessment was done through subjective methods, where a panel of experts was needed to perform the assessment; however, with the development of computer vision techniques, objective methods, such as Breast Analysing Tool © (BAT), proposed by Fitzal *et al.* [33], and Breast Cancer Conservative Treatment Cosmetic Results (BCCT.core) developed at Institute for Systems and Computer Engineering, Technology and Science (INESC TEC)[1], which perform the assessment based on asymmetry measurements, have been used. Currently, in order to use BCCT.core, users must download, install and set-up the software on their computers; these three steps may be considered a burden for some of the users and they also imply that the software will use their computational resources to properly function. On the other hand, fundamental services such as software maintenance (updates and/or upgrades) or support could be difficult in an offline setting. Following the work of Gonçalves *et al.* [42], we propose to move BCCT.core into a web-based application, capable of integrating deep learning models that automatically perform the cosmetic assessment of BCCT.

1.2 Motivation

Breast cancer has physical and psychological impacts on patients [68] and it does not affect only the person who has this disease but also the people near him/her and by consequence, their Quality of Life (QOL). This is one of the main reasons why it is so important to develop an approach to improve the quality of the treatment and the quality of life of every person involved [68, 79]. There are some technologies, like BAT and BCCT.core [17, 33] that can help to fight this problem but they have some limitations, even though the use of technology is growing up in all areas of our society, and in health care is not an exception [58, 108], these technologies can create some difficulties to the users. Currently, to use BCCT.core, users must download, install and set-up the software on their computers; these three steps may be considered a burden for some of the users. On the other hand, fundamental services such as software maintenance or support could be difficult in an offline setting. To overcome these issues and taking into account that most of the healthcare institutions have an Internet connection, we aim to study the best approaches to move BCCT.core into a web-based application, capable of integrating deep learning models (developed by the group) that automatically perform the cosmetic assessment of BCCT. We strongly believe that it will be a great asset that will contribute a lot for the diagnosis, treatment and research for a disease which has a huge impact in our society [100], and by consequence will raise the quality of life of every person involved in this process. Moreover, it will be a great help to all the specialists and institutions that are in charging of taking care of this disease.

1.3 Objectives

Nowadays, these conservative techniques can help to deal with breast cancer, improving the clinical treatment for the patients and help the physicians during the diagnosis period. In the past, this assessment was done through subjective methods, where a panel of experts was needed to perform the assessment; however, with the development of computer vision techniques, objective methods, such as BAT© [33] and BCCT.core [17], which perform the assessment based on asymmetry measurements, have been used. However, none of these two approaches is considered a gold standard, leaving, thus, space for further investigation. Recently, results obtained by Gonçalves *et al.* on breast keypoint detection (essential for the asymmetry measurements) have shown that deep learning algorithms could be part of the answer to reaching a gold-standard method for the aesthetic assessment of breast cancer surgery outcomes [42, 101]. On the other hand, it is important to develop a novel application capable of integrating such deep learning models and accessible from the web, without the need for software installation or in-house maintenance. The main goal of this project book is to create a fully-functional web-based application that allows the integration and training of deep learning algorithms for the aesthetic assessment of BCCT while showing clinical users an intuitive interface that gives them the option to manage their BCCT patient databases and to save records for clinical or investigation purposes.

1.4 Outline

Besides Introduction, this book contains seven more chapters.
Chapter 2 describes the study of important topics approached in this project book. **Chapter** 3 presents the technologies that are needed to understand the motivation behind this project.
Chapter 4 shows all the data collected during ours requirements gathering.
Chapter 5 talks about the workflow and explains the reason behind the use of some tools chosen for us.
Chapter 6 discusses some techniques used in machine learning deployment and shows our performance results.
Chapter 7 presents all the decisions made by us during the development of this project.
Chapter 8 concludes this project book and presents new technologies to future work.

Chapter 2

Background

This chapter contains an overview of fundamental topics such as cancer, web development, databases and machine learning.

2.1 Cancer

Cancer is a cluttered growth of cells, usually derived from a single abnormal cell who had mutations, with the ability to multiply without control in other cell tissues without dying. This type of cells has the capacity of propagation in circulatory and lymphatic systems originating, thus, metastasis. This phenomenon is called invasive cancer cells [45, 109]. The majority of the cancers are originated from epithelial cells and are called carcinomas. Although not being a contagious disease, the number of people who have cancer is growing year after year, a consequence of an increase in population longevity, being age the main risk factor [100]. The incidence of the various types of cancer change with the gender and age; the most common in men are the colorectum, lung, stomach, prostate and liver, while among women are the breast, lung, colorectum, cervix and stomach. Medicine is developing so fast that it is possible to detect and treat cancer efficiently. Therefore, the number of people dying because of cancer is decreasing [39, 73, 100]. Most cancers are named after the cells that give rise to them. For example, if the cells which originated the cancer are from the breast, the disease caused by them will be called breast cancer. If these breast cancer cells spread in the body from a distance, metastasising the lungs, for example, the cells we will find there are breast cancer cells and not lung cancer cells. These non-pulmonary metastases will be treated as breast cancer rather than as lung cancer.

2.1.1 An Overview of Breast Cancer

Breast cancer is one of the most common and deathly types of cancer worldwide. It is originated on the breast, most frequently from the ductal or the lobular carcinomas that supply the ducts with milk [45, 107]. This type of cancer is more common in women [73], but it can appear in men, although it is rare. The most common types of breast cancer are [70]:

- Invasive ductal carcinoma (IDC): Cancer cells grow outside the ducts into other parts of the breast tissue.
- Invasive lobular carcinoma (ILC): Cancer cells spread from the lobules to the breast tissues that are close by.
- Ductal carcinoma in situ (DCIS): Considered the earliest stage of breast cancer, DCIS is non-invasive and it is originated inside a milk duct in the breast.
- Lobular Carcinoma in Situ (LCIS): It is not considered true cancer but it increases the risk of developing cancer during a lifetime.
- Inflammatory breast cancer (IBC): It is different from other types of breast cancer because it is rare (accounts for only 1-5% of all breast cancers). The treatment and the symptoms are different (e.g., redness-like inflammation caused by cancer cells who are blocking lymph vessels in the skin).

2.1.2 Breast Cancer Diagnosis

According to the American Cancer Society, when breast cancer is detected early and is in the localized stage, the 5-year relative survival rate is high [45, 96, 100]; this is why it is so important to diagnose as fast as possible. Breast cancer cells generally create a tumour that can be found on an x-ray as a lump. Any breast lump or change needs to be checked by a doctor to verify if it is benign or malignant (cancer) and to find the best treatment approach. Although most of them are benign, they can be considered an indicator of the probability of getting breast cancer in the future. A brief explanation about the most usual breast cancer diagnostic exams is presented below [54]:

- Breast Self-Exam (BSE): This is an exam in which women do self palpation on the breast to attempt to discover anomalies or to see if the appearance of the breast has suffered changes: if this happens, they should report to their physician [16, 76].
- Clinical Breast Examination (CBE): It is like BSE but the palpation is done by a clinician. One of the best advantages is that CBE can be very efficient in the detection of potentially lethal breast cancers while being simple and inexpensive [76].
- Breast Mammography: It is important in the early diagnosis of breast cancer and can detect the disease before any changes or symptoms in clinical examination appear. Mammography, based in x-ray technology, is one of the most common techniques used, taking into account the fact that this type of diagnosis is linked with many benefits and can decrease (in about 19%) breast cancer mortality [54, 109, 112].

- Ultrasound: This technique is characterised by the use of high-frequency sound waves that will be differently reflected by the breast, generating, thus, diagnostic quality images [54, 83]. One of the main advantages of ultrasound is the fact that it does not use radiation, being very useful for diagnosis in pregnant or young women [4].
- Breast Magnetic Resonance Imaging (MRI): This technique is based on radio frequency wave technology that works on a strong magnetic field. Its main goal is to obtain images from various anatomic plans [54]. This way, it is possible to perform an accurate medical diagnosis where it is possible to show, with high resolution, organs and tissues of the human body. With MRI, clinicians can access important information such as the stage of breast cancer, evaluation of microcalcifications or the presence of residual tumour in patients who underwent surgery [93].

2.1.3 Breast Cancer Treatments

Breast cancer treatments imply a joint work between many specialists to try to identify the best treatments to do in different cases of breast cancer disease. Treatment depends on many things such as the combination of socioeconomic, lifestyle factors, tumour characteristics, age of the patient, pre or post-menopausal state and stage of breast cancer [50, 59, 69]. What will determine the type of treatment is, in fact, the combined interaction of these factors. Usually, the first approach is characterised by breast surgery. The surgical procedure used for the treatment of breast cancer generally affects the breast and armpit. The most common breast surgery types are:

- Lumpectomy: Cancerous tissue and a part of the breast are removed leaving the remaining breast unaffected. Usually, the surgeon also removes the lymph nodes from the armpit. In the case of conservative surgery (also called tumorectomy or quadrantectomy), the woman will be subjected to subsequent radiotherapy [31, 32].
- Mastectomy: The entire breast is removed and, usually, the surgeon also removes the lymph nodes from the armpit. If the woman wishes to do so, and her clinical case permits, in the same surgical procedure as the mastectomy, breast reconstruction may be performed immediately by a plastic surgeon [59]. The most appropriate type of reconstruction varies according to the woman's age, physiognomy, the type of surgical treatment used for breast cancer: breast implants or tissue from another part of the woman's body may be used [63].

These two techniques are known as Breast Cancer Conservative Treatment (BCCT) and Breast Cancer Surgery (BCS) [31, 63]. In this book, we will focus on the BCCT. Figure 2.1 shows a scheme of the cycle of care of a breast cancer patient.

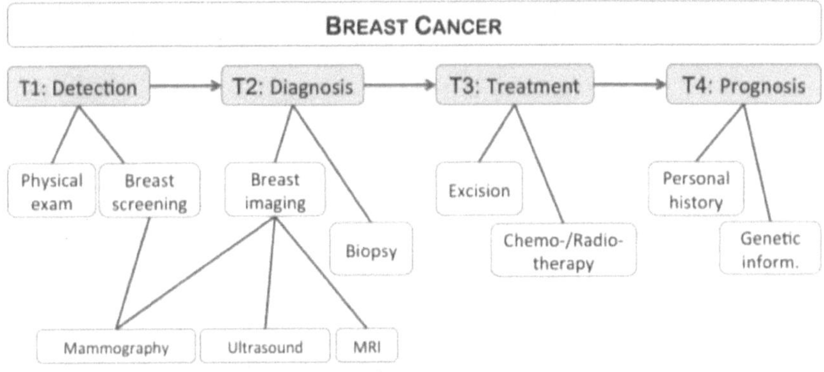

Figure 2.1: Breast Cancer Cycle of Care, from [107].

2.2 Web Development

2.2.1 History

The number of people that uses the Internet, or that has access to it is increasing year after year [51, 89]. We can say that this number will still be growing up in the next years because the Internet has assumed an important role in our lives that we can not deny. This is one of the biggest technological inventions in human history and, in an epoch where every minute is important, we can have global access to the information that we need in seconds. Initially, the objectives were solely military and, for a while, this form of connection between computers was exclusive to the U.S. military. Then, in September of 1969, the Advanced Research Projects Agency (ARPA) developed the Advanced Research Projects Agency Network (ARPANET) [19]. In the late 1970s, protocols that would allow communication between computers and networks regardless of the equipment or software used began to be developed. In addition to this, the Transmission Control Protocol (TCP) and Internet Protocol (IP) were adopted, which also contributed greatly to this development. IP allows communication between computers and TCP ensures greater security in data transmission, among other features. From then on the Internet has grown steadily in terms of users [67].

2.2.2 Overview

Web development can take many meanings depending on the context. In practice, this is the work that is needed to do when someone wants to create a website. Also, it is important to understand that there are many areas involved like graphic designing, programming or software engineering [22]. This world has changed a lot in the last years. For instance, a small number of sites are being created from scratch; instead, actually, a huge advantage for web developers is the existence of many sophisticated frameworks that help on this creation. The next subsection talks more about them and their most important aspects.

2.2.3 Frameworks

According to [29, 57], a framework can be defined as a reusable design of all or part of a system that is represented by a set of abstract classes and the way their instances interact. Therefore it can also be seen as a set of reusable tools or an object-oriented technique that helps the developer to create an application. Although many programmers need to learn how to use the frameworks, they prefer to use them because they provide a lot of useful resources [37, 57]. Moreover, frameworks are also related to many methodologies that are very helpful to fulfil the requisites of a developer, like fast application development and Agile methodologies [110].

2.2.3.1 Web Application Frameworks

The main purpose of web application frameworks is to help developers on the development of a web application. Many frameworks have been growing in the past years: Ruby on Rails, Zend (written in PHP), CataLyst (written in Perl), Ember (written in JavaScript) or Django (written in Python) [110]. Although there are common functionalities among all these frameworks, some of them may be more appropriate for certain tasks. To talk about frameworks, it is fundamental to talk about the principles and design patterns like:

- "Do not repeat yourself" - that defends the existence of uniqueness in a system and tries to reduce repetition on all of the software [52].
- "Convention over configuration" - which is another methodology that aims to help the developer to reduce the number of decisions without reducing flexibility.

Moreover, these design patterns bring solutions for recurrent problems that the developer can find during the development of the project and may improve the communication between developers through a specific vocabulary [47, 56]. Model-View-Controller (see Figure 2.2) is an example of this and we will explain next:

- Model - helps the developer on the management of the rules and the logic of the application sustaining the data [15, 26, 66].
- View - is a specific interface for the user, i.e., it shows information like tables, diagrams or data from the application to the user, allowing the user to make changes;
- Controller - receives as input the output of the user and transforms the information into logic commands [26, 66].

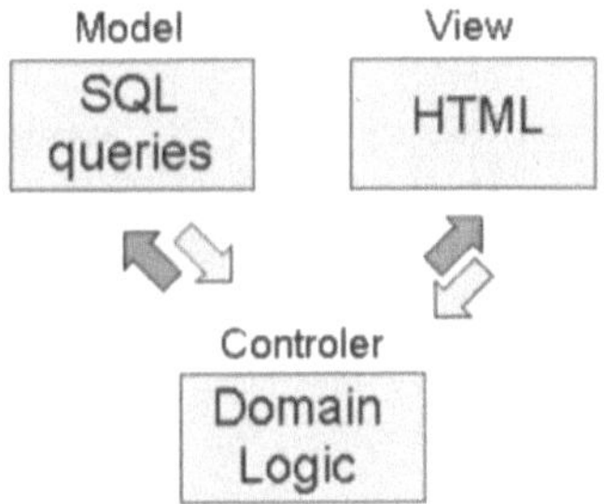

Figure 2.2: Model-View-Controller framework, from [15, 26, 66].

2.3 Databases

2.3.1 History and Overview

A database system is a computerised system to save a set of data. It is very important to think about the database when we want to develop an application because if we will deal with data, the database will have an important role to process and manage all these data. Without, we are not able to manage the application's data in a successful way [60]. These systems have been used a lot in the past years and the history behind this creation had its start in the 1960s. Databases started with the hierarchical and network database management systems. This innovation created a huge revolution on the market and in many companies [43]. Relational Database Management Systems (RDMS) nowadays are extremely important in computer science [8] and with the increase of the size of data sets these systems can not afford so many quantities of data. Therefore we need to find some solutions to this problem. This is where Non-Relational Database Management Systems (NRDMS) come [9].

2.3.2 Relational vs Non-Relational Databases

Relational and non-relational databases were built with different goals. They have specific characteristics that permit us to differentiate between them. Relational databases can be characterised by an Atomicity, Consistency, Isolation and Durability (ACID) principle [44] that aggregates the qualities that should be implemented when we use this type of databases [99]:

- Atomicity - Requires that every operation has to be done without failures. If not, that operation can not be successfully done.
- Consistency - Requires the database to be consistent along with all the operations.
- Isolation - Requires that the transactions between the server and the client have to be done independently from the other clients who share the same database.

- Durability - Requires that when an operation is done, it has to be maintained unchanged.

Examples of relational databases are Oracle[1], MySQL[2], Microsoft SQL Server[3], PostgreSQL[4]. On the other hand, there are some NRDMS based on the Basically Available, Soft state, Eventual consistency (BASE) theorem [86] and Consistency, Availability and Partition Tolerance (CAP) theorem [41]. We can say that a system follows the CAP theorem if the distributed computer system cannot guarantee all three properties simultaneously: Consistency (explained above), Availability and Partition tolerance [40, 41]:

- Availability - The database always returns a value as long as at least one server is running - even if it is a lagged value.
- Partition tolerance - The system will still work even if communication with the server is temporarily lost. Thus, if there is a communication failure with one node of the distributed network, the other nodes will be able to respond to requests for data queries from customers.

Examples of non-relational databases are Cassandra[5], Redis[6], CouchDB[7], MongoDB[8]. The BASE theorem is defined by the following key characteristics [99]:

- Basically available - The system does not guarantee availability under the CAP theorem.
- Soft state - The state of the system may change over time even without input.
- Possible consistency - The system becomes consistent over time if during this period it does not receive any input.

2.3.3 Performance

Elasticity and scalability are two important factors that define good or bad database performance. Elasticity is the capacity of our database to adapt to the increase of data that we need to store and scalability is the capacity of work that our system can deal with [11, 106]. There are two types of scalability: scaling-up and scaling-out. Undoubtedly, scalability should be thought of in application design time as this is not a feature we can add to our application later. Decisions we make during coding in the early stages of the project dictate the scalability of our application. Scaling-up is a term commonly used to achieve higher performance of our application using the best and fastest hardware. This includes adding more features to our server. Scaling-out is

Database	Number of Operations					
	10	**50**	**100**	**1000**	**10000**	**100000**
MongoDB	8	14	23	138	1085	10201
RavenDB	140	351	539	4730	47459	426505
CouchDB	23	101	196	1819	19508	176098
Cassandra	115	230	354	2385	19758	228096
Hypertable	60	83	103	420	3427	63036
Couchbase	15	22	23	86	811	7244
MS SQL Express	13	23	46	277	1968	17214

Table 2.1: Performance comparison between different types of databases on the read time operation, from [71].

another approach of scalability that is responsible to split the data along many servers increasing the amount of data that we can save in our database [11]. Relational and non-relational databases' performance is not a strict definition because it depends on the types of operation and the type of database that we are dealing with. Read, write, delete and update are some of the operations that we probably need to do when we are using databases and the performance will change from operation to operation [71]. For instance, when we talk about reading operations of some relational databases like Microsoft SQL[9] or Express[10], they show better performance than non-relational databases such as CouchDB or RavenDB[11] (see Table 2.1). On the other hand, when we talk about instantiating a database bucket (a place where the data of our database is saved), we can see that non-relational databases such as MongoDB, RavenDB or CouchDB may show better performance (see Figure 2.3). Non-relational databases (also referred to as NoSQL databases) have many advantages but that does not mean we should use them in all situations. On many systems, we may and should use the relational model. NoSQL is best suited for those systems that have higher storage and performance needs. NoSQL is not meant to replace SQL, but rather to provide yet another alternative to a more flexible database in support of data. Therefore, we may use both solutions for different use-cases. Besides, the most common in successful scalar solutions is the use of a hybrid architecture, taking advantage of the best of the two models.

2.4 Machine Learning

According to Mitchel, the definition of machine learning is “A computer program is said to learn from experience (E) with some class of tasks (T) and a performance measure (P) if its performance at tasks in T as measured by P improves with E” [75] or as Shalev-Shawartz and Ben-David affirm, "the term machine learning refers to the automated detection of meaningful

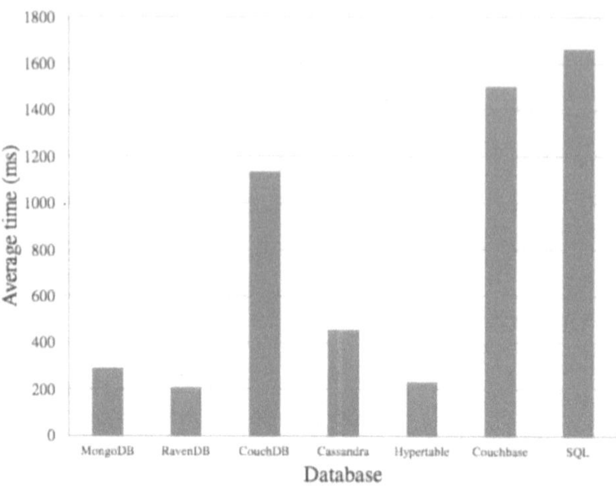

Figure 2.3: Performance comparison between different types of databases on reading a database bucket, from [71].

patterns in data" [97]. In other words, the main goal of machine learning is the creation of models that can take knowledge from observed data, Such knowledge will permit to recognise patterns that will be used for solving future problems. Nowadays, machine learning is used in many ways like spam email detection [94], named-entity recognition [53], machine translation [72], relation extraction [72], information retrieval or sentiment analysis [10]. However, to use it successfully and to have profit out of this tool, it is needed to find the best data set to train our algorithm first [5, 72]. This training data set is known as training dataset and is characterized by a sample of data that are used to fit our model that will extract knowledge from them to be tested in the test dataset. This is the sample of data used to evaluate the model and is used when the model is completely trained.

2.4.1 A Data-Driven Approach

Data is very important when we talk about machine learning. It usually provides the information that we need to solve the given problems and to permit the training of algorithms that will answer new questions that may appear. To choose the best solution it is fundamental to choose or build an appropriate data set. Data mining, the art of exploring the variables on a data set to find some patterns among them [2, 34], gives us the possibility to manipulate and clean the data we use in our processes. Our data has to suffer some modifications such as the removal of outliers, the management of missing values or the reduction of dimensionality to facilitate this processing.

2.4.2 Training Machine Learning Algorithms

Machine learning algorithms can be divided into 3 categories: supervised learning, unsupervised learning and reinforcement learning. Supervised learning refers to the cases when a property (label) is available for a particular data set [18]. Examples of supervised learning algorithms are:

- Regression and Linear Classification - This is the simplest algorithm in machine learning, we have multiple attributes in a matrix with a vector associated with them. The main goal is to find an optimal weight and bias set for these characteristics according to some cost function. Mean Squared Error (MSE) or Mean Absolute Error (MAE) are two examples of these functions and this algorithm is used when we have a huge quantity of characteristics to analyse. Besides, it is also commonly used for numerical variables [3, 28].
- Decision Trees - A decision tree is a model that uses a decision graph and its possible consequences, including chance event outcomes, resource costs, and utility [72].
- Classification Naïve Bayes - Naïve Bayes classifiers are a family of simple probabilistic classifiers based on the application of the Bayes theorem that assumes independence between features [38, 72].
- Support Vector Machines (SVM) - The main goal of this technique is to classify a set of data given as input, find some patterns between them and find the ideal boundary between the different classes taking into account many features. This boundary is given by the support vectors, which will support the classification of a given unseen sample [46, 113].

Unsupervised learning deals with the challenge of finding implicit relationships in a given unlabeled data set (items are not preassigned to specific classes). The main goal of this technique is to find some similarity between objects and create some groups that share identical characteristics. Some of these objects can be different from all the elements of the group; in this specific case, we call it an anomaly [34]. Examples of unsupervised learning algorithms are:

- Clustering Algorithms - It is the task of grouping a set of objects such that those in the same group (cluster) are more similar to each other than those in other groups. This approach uses multiple algorithms, algorithms. A very known example is the k-means that permits this approximation between the objects [38, 55, 72].
- Principal Component Analysis (PCA) - PCA is a statistical procedure that uses an orthogonal transformation to convert a set of possibly correlated observations of variables into a set of linearly uncorrelated variable values called principal components [104].

Reinforcement learning is between these two extremes - there is some form of feedback available for each step or predictive action, but no precise etiquette or error message [105]. This technique is different from all previous tasks because there is no training set, labelled or not, it is inspired in behavioural psychology and the process of acquiring knowledge of the agent, as the algorithms can be called here, occurs from the direct experimentation of the agent's actions in a certain environment. Reinforcement learning is an area of machine learning that investigates how software agents should act in certain environments in order to maximize some notion of cumulative reward [36, 92].

2.4.3 Deep Learning

Deep learning is a specific field of machine learning used in tasks that require a high level of abstraction such as computer vision or speech recognition [64]. It mostly consists of the usage of neural networks with many layers to find patterns in data. Layers are created from many nodes, neurons or computation graphs that can compute information by combining the inputs from the data with learned weights that give importance to the task that the algorithm is learning. The quantity of information that we can extract from our data varies with the number of layers of the neural network, i.e., the deeper the network the higher the amount of information. This is very important when we try to increase our accuracy and precision in finding patterns [7, 64]. A Deep Neural Network (DNN) is a Feed-Forward Neural Network (FFNN) where the data between the nodes goes only in one direction. By consequence, any node is repeated in this process. A Recurrent Neural Network (RNN) is a FFNN that is characterized by using a time twist. Information flows in many directions through time. Also, the information of a specific layer depends on past states and this is why information persists. A Convolutional Neural Network (CNN) is another type of a DNN that is very used in image analysis and recognition [7, 65, 95].

Chapter 3

State of the Art

This chapter explains the technologies that are needed to understand the motivation behind this book project. It focuses on the software that is currently used to perform the aesthetic assessment of BCCT, the availability of commercial solutions, the state of the art algorithms that are behind the aesthetic assessment of BCCT and their future integration into a web application.

3.1 Aesthetic Assessment of Breast Cancer Conservative Treatment (BCCT)

The ubiquity of computer science has greatly boosted research in the most various scientific areas. Medicine has been one of the areas most benefited by the evolution of increasingly accurate and efficient medical procedures that will permit faster and more accurate diagnosis [77]. The evaluation of the result of BCCT is a concrete example of this application. To overcome the limitations of reproducibility and practicality of current subjective methods, recently some innovative computer-assisted systems have been developed such as Breast Cancer Conservative Treatment Cosmetic Results (BCCT.core) [17] and Breast Analysing Tool © (BAT) [33, 61]. The next sections will explore further these software applications.

3.1.1 BAT and BCCT.core Software Applications

BCCT.core introduced the automatic measurement of various indices related to the aesthetic outcome of surgical intervention, making a quick, easy and reproducible evaluation. The measurements are preceded by the automatic location of some reference points (nipples, breast contour and supra-sternal notch) in digital photography. In asymmetry measurements, the colour difference between the treated and untreated breasts and the visibility of the surgical scar are subsequently based on these reference points. At the same time, the set of measurements is automatically converted into a general objective of aesthetic result evaluation, based on an automatic classification algorithm. This algorithm has been trained and optimised to predict the overall aesthetic result. The objective assessment provided by BCCT.core is a summary of the overall aesthetic result, which enables effective comparison between different work teams from any centres [1]. BAT is another important approach used that computes the Breast Symmetry Index (BSI) from digital photographs. The factors used to calculate the BSI are the position of the mammilla regarding the breast border that is saved in the $\text{BSI}_{Mammila}$ and the BSI_{Area} that saves the difference from the area and the circumference from both breasts [61]. The sum of the BSI_{Area} and $\text{BSI}_{Mammila}$ results in the final BSI and the range of this evaluation goes from 0, the best symmetry, to 15, the poorest symmetry (see Equation 3.1).

$$\text{BSI} = \text{BSI}_{Mammila} + \text{BSI}_{Area} \tag{3.1}$$

This method has good accuracy, near 98% [33] in predicting the BSI, becoming a good help in dealing with the evaluation of breast cancer reducing the assessment time [61].

3.2 Deep Learning Algorithms for the Aesthetic Assessment of BCCT

When we talk about the algorithms used on the aesthetic assessment of BCCT we need to talk about Deep Neural Network (DNN) and Convolutional Neural Network (CNN). The state-of-the-art methodology is the result of the combination of two models [101]. The first one, U-Net [90], was used for heatmap regression and refinement to create a representation of the fuzzy localization of the keypoints. The second model uses as input the multiplication of the image by a refined heatmap (i.e., the output of the first model) and employs a VGG16 [88] along with convolutional and fully-connected layers to compute the coordinates keypoints (breast contour, nipples and supra-sternal notch) [101].

3.3 Medical Web Applications

Recently, the number of medical web applications has been growing up very fast with the development of many aspects such as design, protocols or frameworks [89]. There are very recent works about the creation of pre-requisites for developing a successful web application and these requisites depend always on the area of application [24]. Medical web applications have demonstrated their usefulness for both doctors and patients, helping them on the treatment or diagnosis of many diseases. For instance, nowadays, it is possible to avoid the queues at the hospitals with a web application, as reported in [87]: a patient can measure the heart rate at home and doctors can check this variation in a real-time setting. Another example is BCCT.core where the doctors can see the aesthetic changes of breast cancer after surgery with digital photography. To this type of applications to be successful, we need to take care of some issues. Since we are dealing with sensitive information (clinical data), security is one of the most important aspects that we need to take care of [27]. With a medical web application, this information is saved online, so, by consequence, it becomes potentially available to be stolen by other entities that may use this data for malicious purposes. This is the reason why is so important to have protocols and rules that may prevent this problem and give security to the users while using these applications. In the last years, we are assisting an evolution to protect sensitive data from possible outsiders than can use this data for malicious objectives. An example of that is the creation of The European Data Protection Regulation[1]. There are some examples of medical web applications dealing with breast imaging being used like PenRad[2], NovaRad[3], Compass[4]. They became indispensable tools in healthcare treatment.

3.3.1 Designing Interfaces at Medical Web Applications

To design the interfaces we focus in multiple examples of web applications and all are different from each other, these designing interfaces are mostly influenced for the main purpose that each application will be the focus and for their users' needs [78]. These users can differ in many ways, for example, in Portugal the average of medical doctors are more than 50 years old[5], and at the area of cancer, these numbers are very similar[6]. So, we need to adapt and create a simple design interface with the requirements asked by the users that will depend on many variables, like the age or the ability of certain users to work with these technologies. These user needs will be explained with more detail in chapter 4. All of our decisions are based and justified in these results and are according to the preferences of the future users of our project.

3.4 Towards the Integration of Machine and Deep Learning Models in a Web Application

Several services may help on the integration of machine learning algorithms in a web application. It depends on the type of algorithm we want to implement. First, we need to understand our model and find the best approach to use it in our project in the most efficient way. After this step, we need to deploy the web application on a server and create an Application Programming Interface (API) to facilitate access to our model. They are a way to integrate systems, enabling benefits such as data security, ease of exchange between information with different programming languages and monetization of access [20]. Before choosing hosting plans, we have a lot of variety of frameworks in Python for the creation of our API, like Flask[7], Django[8], Pyramid[9] or Falcon[10]. The final decision depends on the specific characteristics of them. All web applications need space on the Internet. This space can be purchased on servers from web hosting companies which offer various types of hosting to their customers and these hosting plans vary according to the space we need for the web application. There are some types of hosting plans:

- Shared Hosting - This type of web hosting simply means that a particular blog or site shares the same server with others. Depending on the capacity of the server, and the popularity of the service provider company, one can host hundreds to thousands of websites or blogs.
- Dedicated Hosting - As the name implies, in this type of hosting, a blog or website will have a fully dedicated server.
- Private Hosting - This type of hosting is a bit more technical and is only possible thanks to a recent technology that is called partitioning technology. In practical terms, there is a physical server with several virtual servers that behave like dedicated servers with their own space.

However, this project will be deployed into an in-house server from Institute for Systems and Computer Engineering, Technology and Science (INESC TEC)[11]. We will talk in more detail about this at Chapter 7.

Chapter 4

Requirements Gathering

This chapter describes all the information collected during the process of requirements gathering and shows how we managed to integrate them into this book project.

4.1 Introduction

When we want to create an application it is important to know how to do it and for who it is; therefore, we need to follow some requirements. Requirements gathering is the process of understanding and identifying the needs that the customer expects to be addressed by the system that will be developed, defining what the software will do. It is the first step in the software development cycle, where the functionalities and scope of the project are defined [49]. Our methodology to assess user requirements, design and development followed several steps:

- Step 1 - Elaboration of a form with questions to be posed to medical doctors specialised in breast reconstruction;
- Step 2 - First interview with a specialist and validation;
- Step 3 - Database design;
- Step 4 - Interface design;
- Step 5 - Definition of main attributes;
- Step 6 - Back-end design;
- Step 7 - Second interview with more specialists of the Champalimaud Foundation[1] in order to get more feedback and validation about the current state of our application;
- Step 8 - Database validation;

- Step 9 - Interface validation;
- Step 10 - Integration with Breast Cancer Conservative Treatment (BCCT) algorithms.

In order to closely meet the users' requirements for Breast Cancer Conservative Treatment Cosmetic Results (BCCT.core), we interviewed Medical Doctor Carlos Mavioso, a specialist in breast aesthetic reconstruction, using a proper form built for this purpose. This form was built taking into consideration good practices used for the development of user interfaces which was validated by Medical Doctor Carlos Mavioso. The objective was to understand the perspective of clinical users regarding some aspects of our future application. Appendix 1 presents the transcript of the interview, validated by the Medical Doctor Carlos Mavioso, where it is possible to see the questions and answers related to the design concerns and database structure.

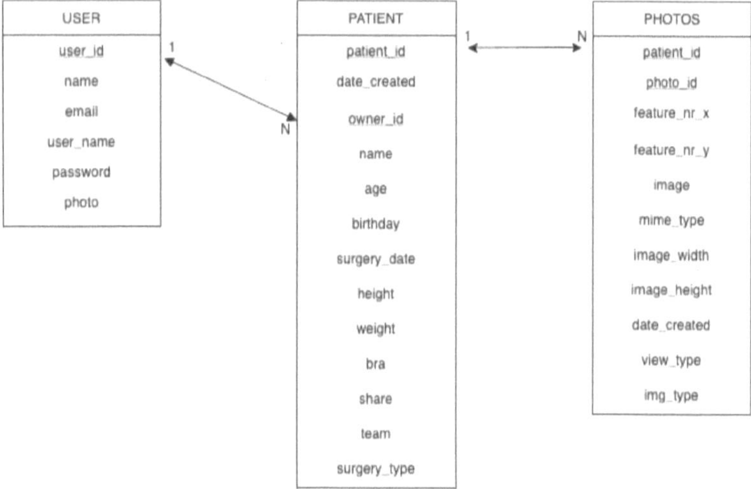

Figure 4.1: Proposed database structure in first iteration.

The second moment of requirements gathering was done during the development of the book project, on a meeting with the Medical Doctors Maria João Cardoso and Carlos Mavioso, members of the clinical team of Champalimaud Foundation, to understand their perspective on some of the already developed aspects of our application. We consider this meeting to be one of the most important phases in our project because it had a huge impact on the rest of the development phase. Our decisions were based on these opinions to make sure that we were developing a web application that will fulfil all the user necessities. Concerning the objective outcomes of these two moments of requirements gathering, we can state that the interview with the Medical Doctor Carlos Mavioso helped us to understand use-cases such as the login system and the best approach to follow with our web application structure. This first moment allowed us to understand the needs and the workflow of this project. Therefore we decided to construct an entire database from scratch and we chose the best tools to use within this project. The structure of our database in the first iteration can be seen in Figure 4.1. We have a Patient entity that contains all the personal data of each patient. We could understand what are the most important attributes to be saved in our database (that were discussed in the meeting with Doctor Carlos Mavioso) and after that, we chose the best approach to save these data paying special attention to performance issues. All the requirements proposed by the doctor was based on the experience with the old version of BCCT.core with the main goal of improving to a new version. The User entity contains all the data regarding each clinical specialist and we link the patients of each specialist by using the first attribute (see Table 4.1) and the second attribute (see Table 4.1) associated to each specialist. The data saved in our database for each user was established after the meeting with the clinical team of the Champalimaud Foundation.

The second moment of requirements gathering with the Champalimaud Foundation clinical team showed us that we would need to add some features that are of utmost importance to improve the usability and the quality of this book project. Taking this feedback into account, we modified the application database by adding a new entity. The Teams entity was added to the database to create a Team associated with each user and their respective Patients. This new entity (Teams) solved one of the problems that were discussed, more precisely, the request to have a function that would allow associating the users by Teams. By associating each user with their respective Team we created the possibility of sharing knowledge and data about Patients with all the members of the same Team. Another important requirement that was asked by the clinical team of the Champalimaud Foundation was the calculation of the difference in days between the photographs and the date of the surgery, a use-case that would improve the analysis of the evaluation of BCCT. To solve this request, we added a new attribute, attribute number 3 (see Table 4.1), to the Photos entity, that will permit the calculation in days of the difference between the date when the photography was taken and the surgery date. This calculation will be presented in the application interface (see Figure 7). The second iteration and the final structure of the database can be seen in Figure 4.2 and Figure 4.3, respectively.

Attribute Number	**Attribute Name**	**Attribute Definition**
1	owner_id	Stores the id of the user
2	user_id	Stores the identification number of the user
3	date_updated	Saves the date when the photography was taken

Table 4.1: New attributes for the Photos entity, that resulted from the second iteration of the process of requirements gathering.

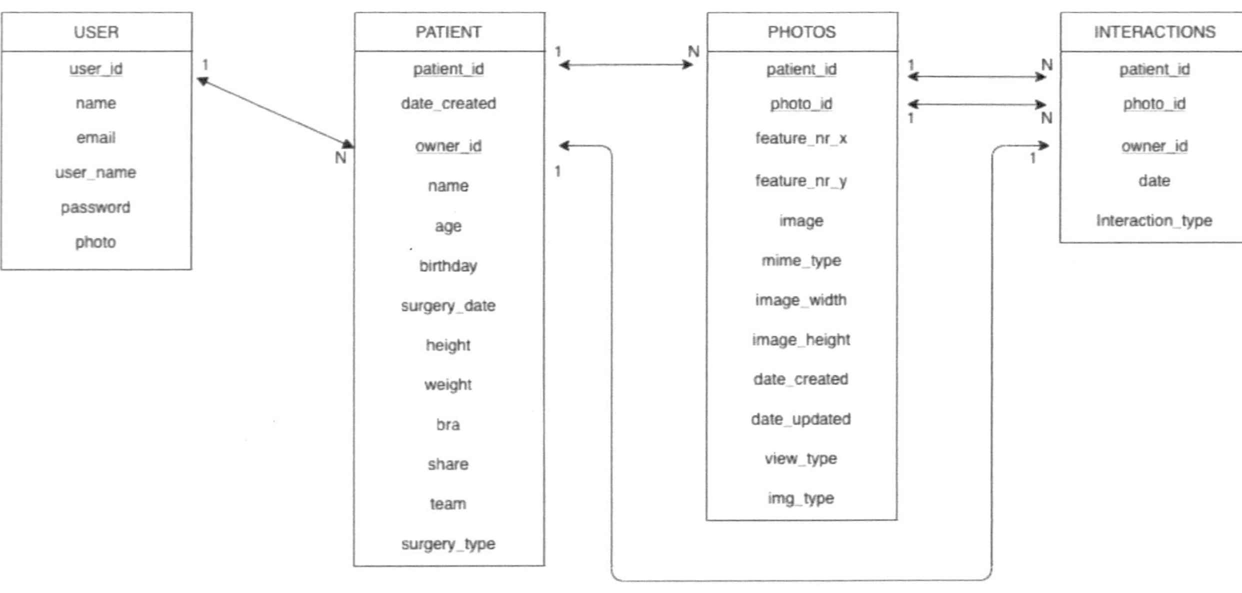

Figure 4.2: Proposed database structure in second iteration.

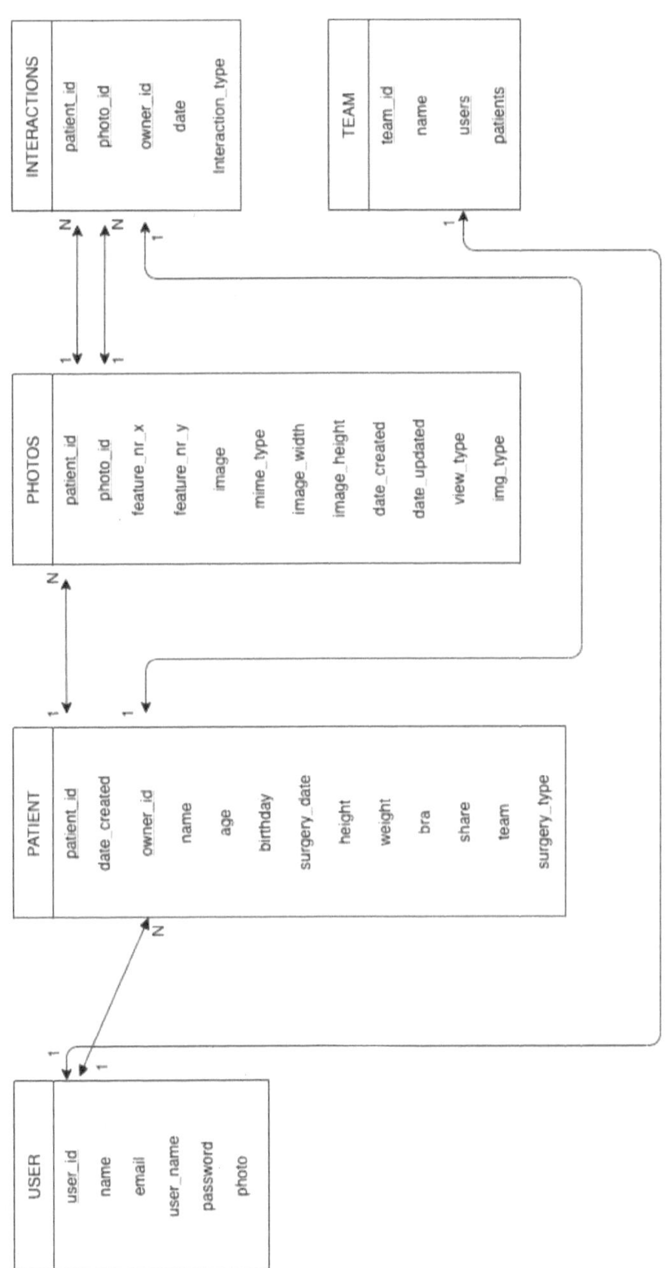

Figure 4.3: Final database structure.

Chapter 5

Web Application Design

This chapter describes the reasons behind the decision of Django and MongoDB as the web framework and database for this project, the implementation of the use-cases and the database performance tests executed.

5.1 An Overview of Django

Django is a Python web framework created in 2003 by a web development team in Lawrence, Kansas and released in July 2005. The name of Django was chosen in honour of a famous jazz guitarist Django Reinhardt. This creation was a huge innovation that opened the possibility to create a web application with a fast and clean design without doing with it from scratch [48]. Based on the previous work by Gonçalves *et al.* [42] we decided to keep this project in Python because it facilitates the interaction with the algorithms and the preliminary work did before. Django is so user-friendly, that a login system can be easily implemented in a short time. Moreover, the use of Django facilitates the interaction with the deep learning models implemented in Python. This framework supports the REST-Ful Application Programming Interface (API) and a built-in user API model for authorization and authentication that provides the developer with a system of *admin-login* (see Table 5.1) that can handle important needs such as permissions or users accounts associated with our project. Also, Django supports HTML output when this format is requested. This type of pages allows developers to navigate more easily and to execute GET and POST commands simply. Django can communicate with several types of databases such as PostgreSQL[1], Oracle[2], MySQL[3], SQLite[4] or MongoDB[5]. It allows the rendering of templates, tables and automatic forms. Besides, functions such as creating tables or indexes can be done with a single command [35, 48]. It is important to take into account that during this process, we were dealing with sensible medical data, so, it was fundamental to pay attention to security issues. Because of this, we have chosen Django since it is already prepared for several attacks like Injection [103], XSS [103], CSRF [103] or Clickjacking [103]. Another important feature of Django is its big community of users. Thanks to this community we can easily search for the tasks that we aim to fulfil while having access to detailed documentation online. Based on these advantages, we have chosen Django. We consider it to be the framework that has the features that were useful for the development of this book project.

5.2 Implementation of the Use-Cases

5.2.1 Login System

We started by implementing a simple login system (see Figure 5.1) that permits the user to register an account with username and password (see Figure 5.1). After that, we used the Allauth[6] Python library that is integrated with Django to allow the use of social media accounts to perform the login. This library separates the local and social networks authentication and permits the use of the API of many social accounts such as Facebook, Twitter or Google as accounts in our login system. To be possible to the user to do a login with their social networks accounts we needed to create an app to use the API of each social network and fill all the information that they need to get access to the App Identification Number (ID) and the Secret Key that will be used on the side of Django Admin Configuration. Using the Django superuser created before, we used the admin console to change our site "example.com" with our private URL. After this stage, we went to the Social Applications field on Django administration to fill with the App ID and Secret Key that we have received before and now we can log in with some social networks that we have already chosen. Both App ID and Secret Key are dependent on each Social Network.

5.2.2 Image Uploading and Processing System

Django gives to the users some structures that are very helpful to construct their models. In this project, we have some of them but we select three that are more relevant. We used three models that are represented and explained with more detail in Table 5.2. With them, we can define some attributes that were chosen before. These models represent their respective entity in our database and after their implementation, we can use them to fulfil our use-cases. Every model has a primary key that links to the other models (see Figure 4.3). Each model structure in Django has some types of attributes defined by default. For example, when we want to specify a field with some attribute type we just need to give a name to our attribute and specify their model type.

5.2.2.1 Store Images in Django

Sometimes, these default approaches can create some problems when we want to do something different with our structure. When we created the model (see Attribute 3 in Table 5.2), we tested our web application and we were only able to upload one image at a time. To solve this problem, we changed our model (see Attribute 2 in Table 5.2) and we updated our model by changing the type field we were using. We changed from model number 1 to model number 2 (see Table 5.3). The reason behind this change was the fact that Django models do not interact directly with the input data from the HTML page. Consequently, we need to use Django Forms. We can see these forms like a link between the input data from HTML to our model. Forms in Django permit the migration of our input data to our model. To update multiple images at once we used an attribute from Django forms, a system of files, this field can read multiple images from the input and save them in a list of files. On the views' section (which process and manipulate all the data and deal with requests from and to the template), we read all the images in our list of files one by one and with some queries that Django provide, we access to the ID of each patient and save all the images to our database. Besides, each of them is associated with the Variable 2 (see Table 5.6). After that, we could read all the images updated by the users and save them with the respective ID of each patient, to know what are the images that belong to each patient.

5.2.2.2 Extracting Images Information

Also regarding the images, we save the metadata in their database. This metadata, also known as Exchangeable Image File Format, or just EXIF, is a specification that allows manufacturers of digital cameras and also cell phones or other camera devices to record information about the technical conditions or settings at the time of capture with the file of the photo. Therefore, in each photo, the camera automatically records how, when and where the image was recorded. This metadata contains information such as the brand and model name of the camera, the dimensions of the photo, the type of the photo, among others. To extract this data from the images we use the Python library Exiftool[7]. When we read a new image we access to this data and save them with the image in the respective entity. To access all the images of the patients without issues, we used a new variable (see Variable 2 in Table 5.6), for each image to be distinct from the other images. For the first image we give this attribute the value of one, for the second image we give this attribute the value of two, and so on. When we try to access images from each patient in our database we have the issue that every image has the same primary key of their respective patient and we can not differentiate each image they are. With Variable 2 (see in Table 5.6), associated to each image, we can solve the problem of access to all the images of each patient, because when we search for that variable that we created at the moment we saved our image in the database, we will find different values for every image that we have and now, it is possible to make the distinction between them. With this, we can create multiple patients associated with multiple images but if we want to update or add more images later we need to create a new solution.

5.2.2.3 Updating Images Information

To solve this issue, we created two update functions to access to all data of the patients and their images. The first update function deals with data to be updated in the second model represented in Table 5.2. We used the UpdateView from Django that permits the users to update all fields of our respective model and saved it instantly on our database. Regarding the second update function, when we update a new image, the first image will be deleted and all data associated with it will disappear. To perform this sensitive operation, the users must type the image ID before the update operation. After this confirmation, we access to the ID of each image and, using queries provided by Django, we delete the first image in our database and we save the new image in our database with the respective value saved in the Variable 2 (see Table 5.6). This variable is returned by a count query that counts all the images that are associated with the Patient that we are updating.

5.2.3 Sharing a Patient

As stated in chapter 4, we acknowledged that one important feature of our Web Application would be to permit users to share patients with other users. To guarantee the security in this operation we only allow the owner of the patient to decide with whom he wants to share the user. For that, we give each patient an owner that will be saved at the fourth variable (see Table 5.6), that represents the ID of the owner. We save this field in a string, Variable 5 (see Table 5.6), which saves all the ID's of the users who have access to that patient. Parallelly to the creation of this feature, we created a view where the users could see all their patients and we added two buttons: one to create patients and another to share the patient ID with other users. To access the shared patients, the users need to search for the ID of the patient. In the back-end, we check if the ID of this user is authorised to access that patient by checking if this ID is saved on the correspondent field (variable number 5 at Table 5.6) in our Patient entity. If it is saved, we permit the access; otherwise, we send an alert to the user stating that he does not have permissions to access to that patient. To guarantee that the user which we shared our patient with can not share the patient again with other users we check if the owner id is the same as the currently logged user. If a user has all permissions to access a certain patient he can make all the operations as if that patient belongs to him, except sharing the patient with other users, as we mentioned before.

Name	**Provider**
Facebook Login	Facebook
Google Login	Google
Twitter Login	Twitter

Table 5.1: Social media accounts used to perform the login.

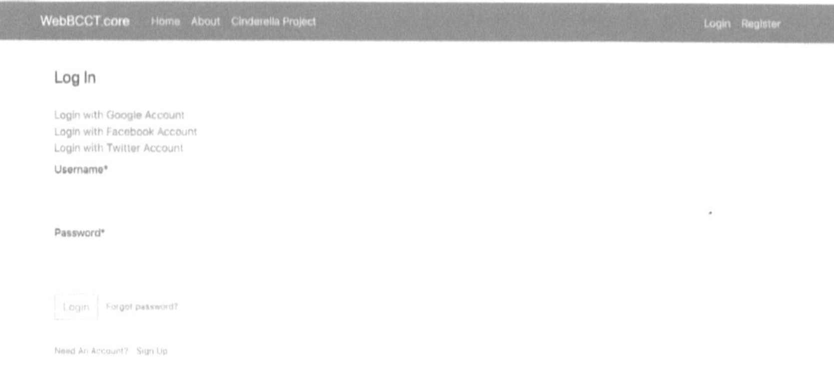

Figure 5.1: Login system implemented with Django.

5.2.4 Team Sharing

Since most of the specialists in this specific area work together (in teams), the Team Sharing use-case is an important function to implement (see chapter 4). This function allows users to share their patients and data with all the members of their team. To implement this, we changed our database structure by adding a new entity to save the data linked with our teams that are constituted by the Variable 6, Variable 1, Variable 7 and Variable 8 (see Table 5.6). Following the workflow of the features that we created before, we start to create our Team model and its respective structure. Every Team has a unique ID to guarantee that we do not have problems with teams that share the same name. Only the administrators of the teams can create and add new users to the teams.

5.2.4.1 Advantages of Team Sharing

The user has the possibility of sharing their patients with all the members of their team and all team members will be able to make modifications in all the patients that belong to the same team. After the user shares the patient with the team, the patients are associated with the team ID to guarantee that each patient belongs to only one team. Before presenting all the team patients to the users, we ask them the team ID that they want to search and we make a queryset to our database by searching for the patients with the specific team ID. This way we have access to all the data of the patients available. To guarantee that members of others teams do not have access to the important data from patients of teams that they do not belong, we verify if the user ID is saved in our team, searching by the ID of the user in our Variable 9 (see Table 5.6), that is used to store all the members that can have access to the data of their team. Depending on this verification, we will decide if the user can have access to this data or not.

Models	Name	Function
1	User	Stores all information regarding to the Users
2	Patient	Stores all information regarding to the Patients
3	PatientImages	Stores all information regarding to the images of Patients
4	Interactions	Stores the interactions done for each user in Patients
5	Teams	Stores all information regarding to the teams that each user belongs

Table 5.2: Models in the database.

Types/Structures	Name	Function
1	model.ImagesField	Stores one object image for variable
2	model.FileField	Stores a list of files for variable

Table 5.3: Model types and structures in our database.

5.3 Choosing the Database Technology

To choose a database we have to think of several details. First, we need to understand our needs and after that, we need to analyse the performance of both types of databases dealing with them. In this project, we assume that we will be dealing with big datasets and that these datasets will have huge quantities of images. Therefore we have chosen MongoDB. In MongoDB, documents are grouped into collections. A set of collections forms a database. MongoDB allows our database to be replicated to other servers, thus increasing the availability of our information (i.e., replication) [6, 84]. Moreover, it is easy to use and manipulate MongoDB databases with Django. This ability allows each server to have a copy of the data and will increase the performance of MongoDB. Besides, it uses replication and scaling-out that permits a good performance on handling large datasets with a big number of requests [60]. MongoDB was created to be easy to manipulate. It is a document-based database in JSON format, so, unlike a relational database, it has no restriction or the need to have the tables and columns previously created, thus, allowing a document to represent all the information we need, with all the data we want. Another advantage of this database is that it is a flexible data model and we are not limited to a defined structure in our schema [6, 84]. Based on these advantages, we decided to choose MongoDB as the database to be implemented in this book project.

5.4 MongoDB Testing Performance

To understand the performance of our MongoDB database we used Yahoo! Cloud Serving Benchmark (YCSB)[8] to study its behaviour with many types of operations and data [23]. This is an open-source framework that permits the comparison performance of services in the cloud data. This performance study was extremely important to understand how MongoDB will deal with our data. YCSB enables the testing of different databases and their comparison. For instance, on the same hardware configuration, multiple databases can be installed and tested over a similar load scenario. Therefore databases' performances can be compared [23]. YCSB works in a similar way to a system who offers online read and write data access (*e.g.*, an user who wants to load a page of a web application). YCSB uses Java to create and process all different types of workloads [23, 62]. A workload is a file that will execute operations in our database. To implement this testing framework, we installed and set up our system test and we choose the appropriate workloads to our application conditions. The main criterion to select the workloads was to pick the ones which to have similar data and working conditions as the web application developed under the scope of this book. We then evaluated the MongoDB performance with this data. Table 5.4 presents the characteristics of the server and Table 5.5 presents the Mongo DB database that we used to run the performance tests.

Processor	Intel(R) Xeon(R) CPU E5-2665 0 @ 2.40GHz
Operative System (OS)	(Linux) Ubuntu 18.04.4 LTS
Random Access Memory	16GB
Storage	96.85GB

Table 5.4: Server Characteristics.

MongoDB shell version	v4.2.3
MongoDB server version	v4.2.3

Table 5.5: Database Characteristics.

We chose Workload C (i.e., read operations only), Workload D (i.e., read operations, but the majority is the insertion of new records in the database) and Workload F (i.e., read, update and write a record in the database). We discarded Workload A and Workload B because the type of data that they have is not the most appropriate to use with our project. By default, YCSB generates workloads that deal with only 1000 records, but the user may change this value to a number that better fits real-world conditions. During our performance tests, we set the number of records to 100 million. This is done by setting the first parameter (see Table 5.7) to the value of 100 million. To be able to load this entire process we chose some runtime parameters to improve our time process like the number of threads. By default, YCSB uses only one but we can add additional threads by a process, with this, we accelerate the process by increasing the number of operations by threads. The final step was to load the data and this phase is divided into two parts. The first one, loading phase which selects the data that will be inserted and processed, the second one is the transactions phase which will define what type of operations will be executed with the data set. To have access to all statistics of the operation, like a time-series that was very useful to construct all the graphics that show the performance behaviour we specify the field of the second variable (see Table 5.7) with the property of timeseries. Therefore we processed the results and built the graphics presented below.

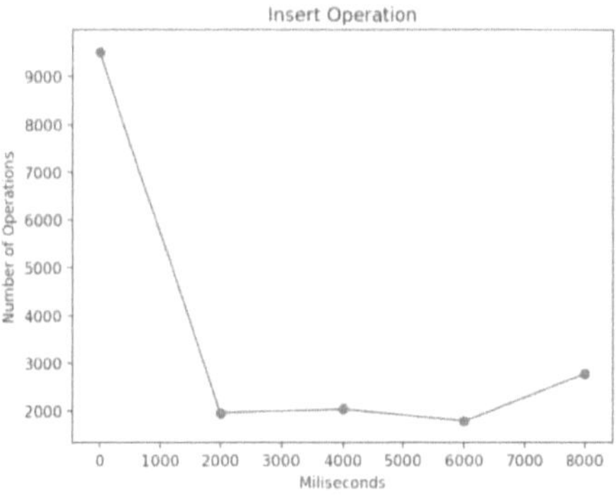

Figure 5.2: Insert Operation in Workload D.

The graphic in Figure 5.2 shows the performance of MongoDB dealing with insert operations, one example of this operation is when someone updates a user or a patient status and tries to access to this information. MongoDB starts to insert a huge number of records, near 9500 records and this number will decrease and maintains the same along all the process, doing an average of 2137 operations per 2 seconds.

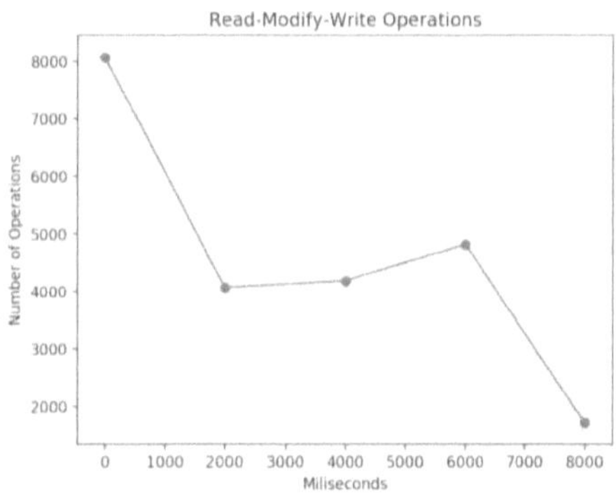

Figure 5.3: Read-Modify-Insert Operations in Workload F.

The majority of operations is focused on reading and modifying patient data. To simulate these conditions, we choose the Workload F because it is the workload that represents best the operations of reading, modifying and writing in our database (see Figure 5.3). The number of operations starts near 8000 operations and will decrease to 2000 operations during all the process. Even though this number is not constant, we can conclude that with MongoDB we have a better performance when compared with a SQL-based database [71].

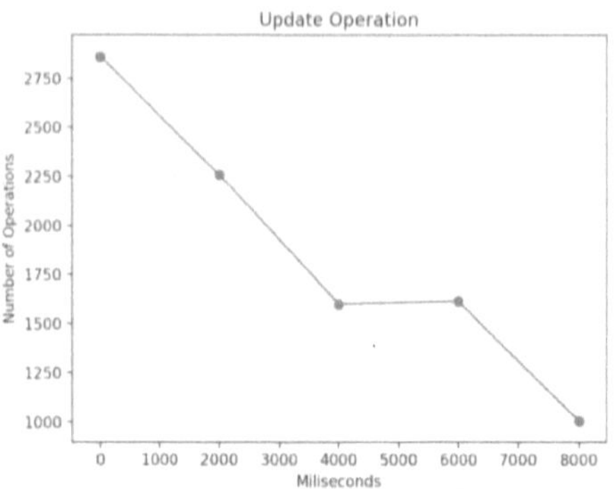

Figure 5.4: Update Operation in Workload F.

Figure 5.5 shows a comparison between the update Operation and the Read-Modify-Write data. MongoDB starts doing near 3000 update operations and will decrease to near 1000 operations along all process.

Each workload has its specificities, so it is important to execute them independently, bearing in mind the operations and the data to process. The main goal here is to understand what is the type of data which interacts better with MongoDB and better simulates the data that our web application will process. To assess the quality of this interaction, we choose the read operation in Workloads C, D and F. From Figure 5.5 we can see that MongoDB has the best performance with Workload F, followed by Workload D and Workload C. Since MongoDB performed best with the Workload F, which better simulates the data used in our web application, we can conclude that it is a suitable database option for this work.

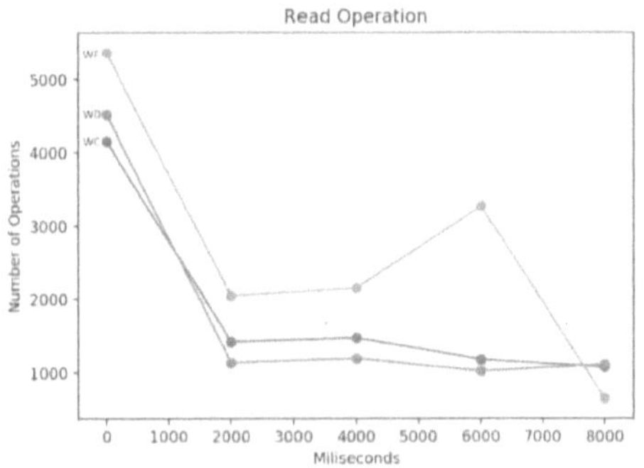

Figure 5.5: Read Operation in Workload C,D and F.

Variables	Name	Function
1	patientID	Stores the patient ID
2	number	Stores the ID of each image
3	imageID	Stores the ID of each patient that an image belongs
4	ownerID	Stores the owner ID of each patient
5	share	Stores the ID of each User which every patient can be shared
6	userID	Stores the ID of each user
7	teamID	Stores the ID of each medical team
8	teamName	Stores the name of each medical team
9	users	Stores the ID's of user in the collection Teams

Table 5.6: Variables used by us.

Variables	Name	Function
1	recordcount	Set the number of records
2	measurementtype	Provides a list with all statistics of the operation

Table 5.7: Variables used by us in the database test performance.

Chapter 6

Machine Learning Deployment

This chapter talks about the techniques that are the most used when we want to develop software with deep learning algorithms running in the background. It starts by defining deployment as the name of the process that permits sharing our work with the world by moving our offline software to online software and it concludes with our study on containers and virtual machines, which are the most common approaches to deploy software nowadays.

6.1 Virtual Machines (VMs) and Containers

Nowadays, the most used technologies for the virtualisation of hardware are VMs and containers. VMs are created from hypervisors which are a type of software that needs an operating system to work. Containers can run without an operating system behind them and they can be executed inside of a VMs [25].

6.1.1 Virtual Machines

Virtual Machines are a type of software in which we can install and execute one or more operating systems. It is the equivalent of running a computer inside another computer. Nowadays, we can easily create a virtual machine. We just need to install the virtual machine software and then create a virtual hard disk to be able to run an entire operating system from it. When we want to use a virtual machine we only need to execute our software and the virtual machine will be executed in a new window. This is only possible because virtual machines work as an organised mix of software with a real machine and during their execution they use a specific quantity of memory. Every machine has its virtual hardware, including memory, processors, network interfaces, hard drives, and the other devices that are part of a standard computer. The reason why they have worst performance compared with a normal computer is by the fact that they are stored in a physical hard-drive and they spend more time to access and process all the information needed to execute all their inner processes. In the VMs universe, we define the host as the operating system that runs on our physical computer and guests as all the other operating systems running inside of virtual machines [102]. There are two types of virtual machines:

- System VMs, which is an environment that permits that many instances of the operating system are running our computer, sharing the physical resources;
- Process VMs, also known as an application VMs, which is the first and the most used type of virtual machine, it is characterised by having processes that have their own address space and give users the possibility of having multiple processes running at the same time [74, 102].

6.1.2 Containers

Containers can be defined as a set of one or more organised processes that are isolated from each other in the system or server [74, 102] that use the host kernel to run virtual environments. This permits that multiple projects can be saved in the same place but with different environments; this approach will permit the better utilisation of hard disks, memory and processors. One example of when we can use containers is when we want to share with other developers our project and they have a different environment configuration. The three most famous used containers are Linux-VServer[1], OpenVz[2], and Linux containers[3] [14] and Docker containers[4]. This book project depends on specific libraries, dependencies and files that we need to use to work efficiently. We consider that containers represent a huge help to solve this problem by creating a single and unique environment for each process [25].

6.2 Virtual Machines *versus* Containers

Although they have some different aspects, it is important to note that these two technologies are complementary. As we mentioned before, and presented at Figure 6.1. The virtualisation is linked with the use of hypervisors to emulate the hardware that permits the users the possibility of using multiple operating systems at the same time, although, this is not always the best option when compared to containers [25, 30]. Generally, when we want to develop some project we need to be aware of our available resources (since they are not unlimited) and we need to choose the best options to efficiently develop our project. For containers, this is a great advantage, because they are executed natively only on the operating system and will bring agility and lightness to the applications [25, 30, 74]. Therefore, we analyse some key aspects of both techniques. When we talk in isolation we are referring to the capacity of a system to maintain two or more processes isolated from each other in the way that they work independently and without the interference of others processes that are being executed at the same time. VMs are better on isolating, and are used when strong security is needed like two projects from two competing developers working on the same server. One of the big differences between containers and VMs is the way that they deal with an operating system. Containers can be customised with some specific configuration to have only the services that they need to run some task. VMs execute an entire operating system. For example, while in a traditional virtualisation system we have an isolated operating system, in the case of containers, we have isolated resources that make use of the native operating system's kernel libraries. This means that we can achieve better performance, compared to virtualisation, and in terms of smaller applications. When we try to execute some project we need to think about how our data will be saved. VMs and containers follow two different approaches. VMs use a virtual hard disk for each user while containers use servers that can be shared by multiple nodes. It is important to note that VMs in the cloud have some behavioural aspects that we need to understand such as their behaviour in situations of load balancing and fault tolerance. In cloud computing, load balancing is the way that the resources are distributed in our environment. When it fails, VMs move resources to another server. On the other hand, in the same situation, containers stop and start the nodes to manage changes. Fault tolerance is another important aspect that can not be discarded: it is defined as the behaviour of our system when an error or a failure occurs during the execution of some task. Both services are similarly dealing with fault tolerance: when it occurs in VMs in the cloud our service will start in another server and if a node in containers fails, they will create a new node for the service that can be possible to work properly again [25, 30, 74].

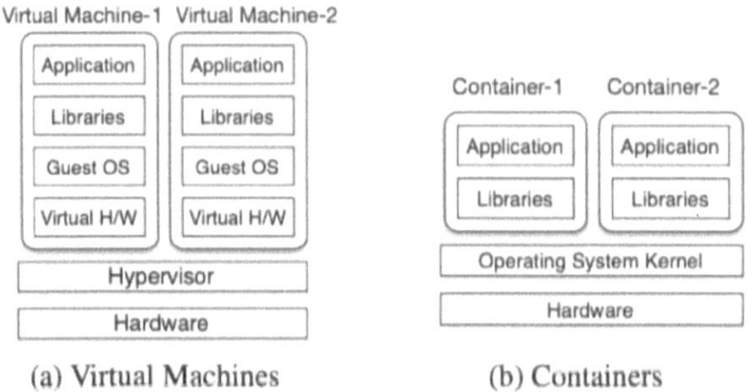

(a) Virtual Machines (b) Containers

Figure 6.1: Containers *versus* Virtual Machines from [98].

6.3 Docker Containers

Docker is an open-source development platform based on the programming language Go from Google [85]. This platform facilitates the management and creation of isolated environments using the technology of containers [21]. Docker has gained a lot of popularity since it allows to "package" an application or system inside a container that can later be run on any machine that has Docker installed. With Docker, it is possible to configure an entire system only one time and then execute in another environment without major issues. This feature is very useful for system administrators. With these features, the deployment time is considerably reduced. Moreover, a solution created in Docker is highly portable.

6.3.1 Deployment with Docker

In this section, we will explain some key aspects that are used in Docker deployment. First, we explain how Dockerfile and *Docker-compose* works and then we analyse all the dependencies related to them [21].

6.3.1.1 The Dockerfile

Docker builds images that are represented in a document called Dockerfile. These images are saved as instructions, so Docker will always know the features that must be installed in the container that we want to run and their order in the building pipeline. These instructions are saved as text in the Dockerfile and they are invoked using the command *"docker build"*. This way, all these instructions will be executed and installed inside the container. When the Docker image is built, a context is launched with a specific path that is used by the container to access the directory system where we have the files that we want to use in our container. The build process is executed by the *"Docker daemon"*. The *"Docker daemon"* is a feature that runs at the host operating system and works like a system of a server-client, where the *"Docker daemon"* has the same role as the server. The best practice to create a container is to start an empty directory as context because, upon creation, the build process sends all the data in context to the *"Docker daemon"*. Moreover, the Docker daemon receives the data context from the Docker Command Line Interface (CLI), which is a command-line tool that creates the bridge of communication with Docker daemon and before sending these data, searches for file *.dockerignore*, that is located at the root directory of our data context. Equivalent to the *.gitignore* file in Git repositories, this file assures that sensitive files or large data are not sent to the *"Docker daemon"*. Therefore, we can avoid adding unnecessary data to the container. To guarantee that this process does not have future errors, a validation of the Dockerfile is executed before the execution of all the instructions by the Docker daemon. If some errors are found in this file, the container will not be created and an alert will be released to the user. One of the multiple advantages of containers is the fast building phase. This happens because every executed command can build a new image which will be stored in the cache of the container. The cache is defined as a storage area where frequently used data or processes are saved for faster future access. This assures time-saving processes and unnecessary use of computer hardware. Also, the Dockerfile has a personalised structure. Conventionally, instructions should be written in uppercase and their arguments should be written in lowercase. More details on the usage of the Dockerfile are explained below.

The piece of code below presents the Dockerfile structure and the instructions used in this project. Table 6.2 organises the type of instructions that we used to build our web application container.

```
FROM python:3.7
ENV PYTHONUNBUFFERED 1
RUN mkdir /code
WORKDIR /code
COPY requirements.txt /code/
RUN pip install -r requirements.txt
COPY . /code/
```

Number	Instruction
1	FROM
2	ENV
3	RUN
4	WORKDIR
5	COPY

Table 6.1: Dockerfile instructions.

- Instruction 1 - This instruction refers to the parent image that will be installed in our container (see Table 6.2). We can repeat this process as many times as the number of images that we need to install in our container. Each time that we execute these instructions, all the data and the states that were saved are cleared. Besides, we can specify the platform we are using. We chose Python 3.7 because it was the environment in which we have been working during this book project. Moreover, it is the Python version that is compatible with all the dependencies and libraries used in this web application.

- Instruction 2 - This instruction creates the environment associated with the variable "PYTHONUNBUFFERED" which will be used in all the instructions that are executed in the building phase. Regarding the usage of this instruction, it is important to notice that we can also use it when we need to create multiple variables associated with the environment that we will create.

- Instruction 3 - This instruction is a command which is used to run any commands in our current image. We can use it in two ways: RUN <command> or RUN ["command", "arg1","arg2"].

- Instruction 4 - This instruction specifies the working directory from where all the instructions will be executed. This instruction can be used multiple times with different working directories paths.

- Instruction 5 - This instruction will add all the data specified in our source path to the filesystem of our container. To match the path for the directory from where we want to copy our data, Docker uses the Go language [85]. When this operation is done, all the directories and files will have a User IDentifier (UID) and Group IDentifier (GID) of 0. Linux uses this UID number to monitor users and check these users records. The term GID stands for Group Identification Number (ID). On Linux, files and directories are organised into groups. The GID of a file is initially inherited from the user who creates the file. Docker permits that we can specify the username or a group name by using the flag *–chown* and specify the parameters associated with it. This is a very important instruction because Docker creates a root filesystem that every container must-have, otherwise the build operation will fail.

6.3.1.2 The *Docker-compose*

The *Docker-compose.yml* file structure is presented below in the piece of code:

```
version: '3'
services:
  mongo:
    image: mongo
    container_name: mongo
    restart: always
    ports:
        - 27018:27017
    environment:
        - MONGO_INITDB_ROOT_USERNAME=jj
        - MONGO_INITDB_ROOT_PASSWORD=password
        - MONGO_INITDB_DATABASE=bcct_bd
  web:
    build: .
    command: bash -c "pip install -r requirements.txt  && python manage.py
        runserver 0.0.0.0:8000"
    volumes:
      - ./:/code
    ports:
      - "8001:8000"
    depends_on:
      - mongo
```

The *Docker-compose* file is written in YAML language. It aims to define services, volumes and networks preferences. YAML language was launched in 2001, inspired by languages such as XML[5], Python[6], C[7], among others. YAML is a recursive acronym that stands for "YAML is not a markup language" and intends to be a human-readable data serialization format, being the reason why is so widely used for configuration files. Data serialization is a process for converting a data structure or an object into a format that can be stored or transferred. It has a simple and

Number	Instruction
1	build
2	command
3	container_name
4	depends_on
5	restart
6	environment
7	image

Table 6.2: *Docker-compose* file Instruction variables.

readable syntax, which can be easily mapped by the most common data types in most high-level languages [13, 80]. We can define *Docker-compose* as a service which has all the configurations needed that a container needs to be able to run. More details about our configuration are explained below.

- Instruction 1 - This instruction receives the path where we want to build our context. In this case, by using the dot, we are informing Docker that we want to build our context in the current directory.
- Instruction 2 - This instruction is very similar to the 'RUN' command used in the Dockerfile. It is possible to provide a list or just a single command to run. Moreover, it is also possible to pass the option "bash -c " to use multiple commands. In this project, the commands provided are used to guarantee that our project runs with the correct libraries defined in the requirements file. After this verification, we start our application with the command "runserver".
- Instruction 3 - This instruction is used to give a specific name to our container rather than a random default name. Every name has to be unique to avoid future errors.
- Instruction 4 - This instruction defines what are the dependencies between services. We selected Mongo because it is related to our database, which will be accessed by the web application.
- Instruction 5 - This instruction decides when the container has to be restarted if some error occurs. We defined as "always" because we need our database to be always running and to grant access to all data that is needed for its proper execution. This command also has some optional arguments, such the delay, that defines how long will we wait for our container to restart again, the maximum number of restart attempts and the maximum number of restart times.
- Instruction 6 - This instruction is very useful to define secret values or specify some values that are used by the host to execute some actions (e.g., a simple login in a database). All the variables used for us in the *Docker-compose* file are linked with the MongoAPI. This way we have access to our data by providing the necessary information to login.

- Instruction 7 - This instruction specifies the image from which we want to build our container (analogous to the Dockerfile). In our case, we only select Mongo image because we have already defined Python as the other image in the Dockerfile.

Docker containers have changed significantly our web application performance. All the changes and results will be discussed in the next section.

6.4 Performance Experiments and Results

Nowadays, taking into account the characteristics of deep learning models, we acknowledge that one of the most challenging aspects is the deployment phase [111]. When we started the development of this project, we understood that the biggest challenge would be to reduce the time of execution of a single request when we wanted to process a single image. Our deep learning model receives a path of an image saved in our database. When the request is launched by the client-side we access to the value saved in variable 1 and variable 2 which are sent in the request (see Table 5.6). We then get their values and run the model with the respective image path. Before the changes in our project architecture, our web application would take twenty seconds to complete the entire process of receiving an image, process it and return the values predicted by our model. To improve this time-consuming request, we decided to use Docker [111, 114]. As we explained before, an important factor here is that the Docker works in layers and these layers are the ones that guarantee the isolation of our application area. This means that with this isolation it is possible to get low consuming-costs and reduced memory space. The deep learning model used in this web application has a considerable dimension to run normally as simple operation and we found several limitations when we wanted to process more than one request. If we increased the number of requests, our container would exit with a memory error. This suggests that we were exceeding the memory of our container when we tried with more than one request because we were loading our model multiple times instead of performing this operation once. To solve this problem, we changed the way the model is loaded to assure that that our free space in memory will not be occupied by redundant operations. To implement this solution we created a global variable that saves the data at the moment of the model loading phase and we use this variable each time we need to call the model. With this change in the project architecture, we can now receive multiple requests at the same time without crashing and overloading our container. The results are presented in Figure 6.2, Figure 6.3 (generated using the macOS Activity Monitor[8]) and Table 6.4.

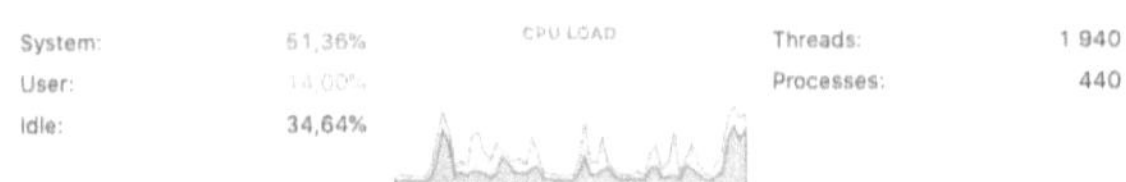

Figure 6.2: Before architecture modifications.

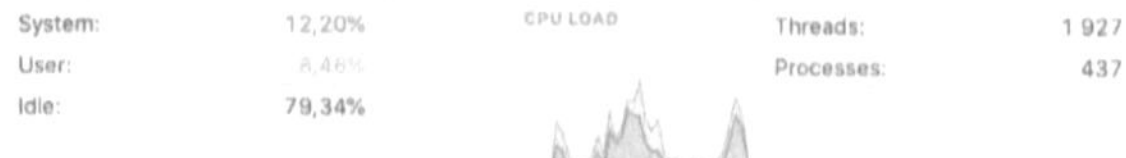

Figure 6.3: After architecture modifications.

Single Request	An average of 20 seconds
Multiple Requests	None

Table 6.3: Before architecture modifications.

Single Request	An average of 5 seconds
Multiple Requests	An average of 30 seconds

Table 6.4: After architecture modifications.

The macOS Activity Monitor (see Figure 6.2 and Figure 6.3) show the processes that are running on the Mac, so we can manage them and see how they affect Mac activity and performance. We performed these tests on a personal computer with the characteristics (presented in Table 6.5) to avoid some issues regarding with login problems in the server where we want to deploy our web application. The CPU panel shows how processes affect the processor activity. The variables used are:

- System: The percentage of CPU capacity currently being used by system processes, which are processes that belong to macOS.
- User: The percentage of CPU capacity currently being used by apps that we have opened or processes that those apps have opened.
- Idle: The percentage of CPU capacity that is not being used.
- Processes: Every instruction that needs to be executed will directly run in a process. The process is controlled by the operating system, and the time that it will take to run depends on the processor availability and the available memory. Also, of course, access permissions to other resources are linked to the process as a whole.
- Threads: Threads resembles the process because each new thread (and everything related to it) will be treated by the operating system in the same way as a process. Threads are useful to save processing-time. But in terms of memory, it is the application's responsibility to control shared access throughout the process.

One of the main goals, when we build an entire application, is to increase the latency of our web application. This is very important because it permits us to have multiple users using our application without having problems with overloading. Increasing the latency of a system means that the number of processes that our CPU has to process will automatically decrease.

System Operative Version	macOS Catalina, Version: 10.15.3
Model	MacBook Pro (Retina, 13-inch, Mid 2014)
Processor	2,6 GHz Dual-Core Intel Core i5
Memory	8 GB 1600 MHz DDR3
Graphics	Intel Iris 1536 MB

Table 6.5: Computer Characteristics.

Analysing these results, lead us to conclude that we are releasing a lot of capacity to run other processes and we can confirm that by the percentage of CPU used after these modifications is significant, we decrease the 'System' from 51% to 12%, the 'User' from 14% to 8% and the 'Idle', that changed more than 50%, from 34% to 79% after these changes. These results say that we decrease the number of processes to execute and by consequence increase the capacity of our CPU to execute more processes. Analysing the results and the execution-time of the requests, we can conclude that we have improved our web application performance in 75% for single requests and 100% for multiple requests.

Chapter 7

User Interface and Experience

This chapter introduces the concept of usability and explains our decisions regarding the user interface and the user experience topics.

7.1 The Importance of Usability

Usability focuses on a set of rules and best practices that measure how users learn and use a product to achieve their goals. It can have different meanings, depending on the area that we are focusing on. Usability also assesses user satisfaction during this process [116]. This area is closely linked with intuition and the ability to communicate a message that is linked to a specific and important action. Nowadays, developers need to know for what kind of user is the application that they are designing. Therefore, they must follow some patterns to make a good user experience in the system. To help with this, some fundamental questions need to be answered [12]:

- Learning: How easy is it for users to perform basic tasks the first time they encounter the design?
- Efficiency: How quickly can they get things done?
- Reminiscence: When users return to the project after a period without interacting with it, how easily can they restore proficiency?
- Errors: How many users make mistakes? How serious are these errors? And how easily can they recover from errors?

These questions have fundamental importance to define a usability framework that will permit the users to easily manipulate the systems and consequently, to increase the probability of success of a project [79, 115]. It is also very important to know how to perform requirements gathering because we need to understand who is our project's audience and the use-cases that we have to address. These issues are very important for the developer too because they provide the answers to some doubts that may appear during the development phase [91, 115]. The final goal is to offer users an application with all the use-cases that they are expecting.

7.2 Explaining Decisions

Most of the implementation and user usability use-cases were based on the requirements defined in chapter 4. These definitions were very important to know how to proceed in every developing stage. Based on these we decided to add some new features to our project.

7.2.1 Patient Share

One of these new features was the patient share, we decided to add a button asking the data that is saved at the variable 1 (see Table 5.6) because it permits the specialist to share a patient with whomever he wants and in a simple way. The specialist only has to open the patient detail page, which is where we show all the information linked with every patient, and the specialist only has to specify the user Identification Number (ID) which he wants to share that patient with. By clicking on the button named 'share', the web application will automatically allow the user which he shared the patient, to access to all data linked with him. This operation has suffered some modifications. In the beginning, we granted all access to the user (read and write operations) which is shared the patient but, after the meeting with Champalimaud Foundation [1] we decided to change these permissions and we only give the read permission, thus removing the permission to change the data that user wanted. The reason to change this was the fact that we need to grant integrity in the data of each patient to avoid that possible external users access to sensitive information and have the possibility of changing some values that are very important the analysis of the evaluation of the Breast Cancer Conservative Treatment (BCCT). By the fact that each patient belongs to a user and a team, by default all the shared patients will be accessible from all the team elements. To avoid adding unnecessary buttons to our template we use the same button for two operations.

7.2.2 Search Button

The search button is used to the specialist search for their patients and patients that are shared with him. To guarantee that our web application is fault-tolerance we verify every possible error that can occur and we send the reason of this error to the user. Fault-tolerance defines a system that can deal with errors along the time. Some possible errors include: the specialist does not have the authorisation needed to have access to the data of a specific patient or the patient ID that the specialist search is wrong or does not exist in our database.

1

7.2.3 The Importance of Patient ID in Sharing Information

We chose the patient ID as input to avoid some possible errors when two patients share the name. Besides, this way is more simple and clean to deal with a unique number like an ID rather than use some redundant variables like the name. In the same logic, we added a button that enables the specialist to search all the patients of his/her team. To create a team we need to follow some security rules because in this case, one user will have access to all the information that the users of the same team will share. Django permits to give some specific roles to a user at the time of the creation like the *admin-user*. The *admin-user* in Django has more privileges than all the other normal users and we used this module to create teams. Each team only can be created by on *admin-user* and this user will be responsible for adding elements to the team which he is the owner. We create two different templates for each type of user.

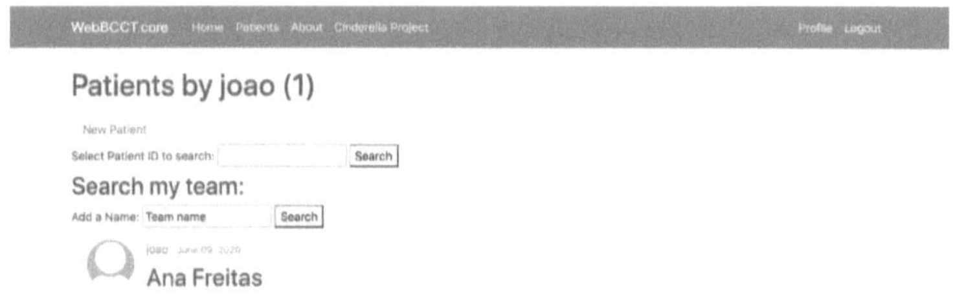

Figure 7.1: Normal User view.

The *admin-user* will have one additional button that permits the creation of a new team and permits to add a new user to the team.

7.2.4 Team Sharing

To perform this operation, we create a new template with two different options to select, first one we allow creating a new team only by asking for the team name that the user wants to create. Every time the user wants to create a new team we check all the names that are already saved in our database and the app will check the availability of this name to create a new team. If this name is in our database we prompt an error message saying that the user needs to use another team name because this one is already in use. The second one is to add a user to the team by the respective team name that the user wants to add. Here, we ask the user ID to add and the app will save in our database all the users that have permission to access to the data team. To check every possible error, if a user exits and is saved in our database or if a user has

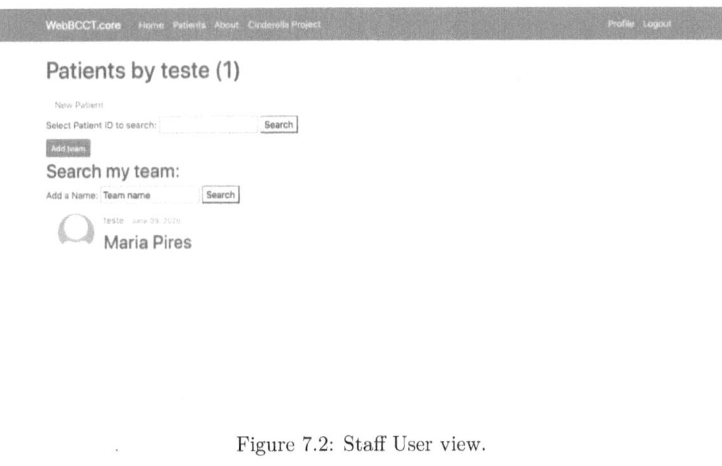

Figure 7.2: Staff User view.

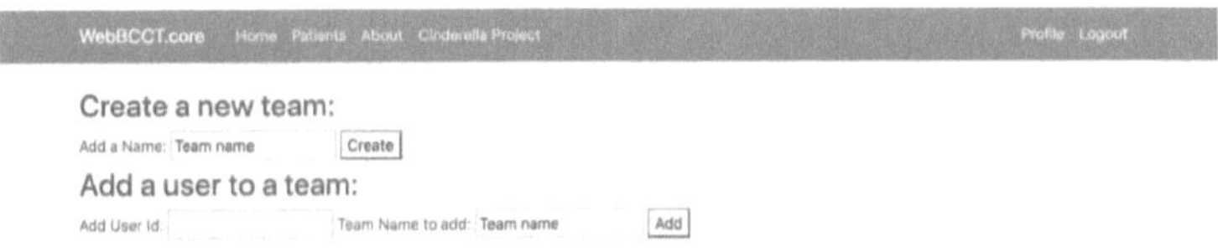

Figure 7.3: User team creation view.

already been added to the team the app will return a message to the user when it occurs. The importance of sharing data and knowledge about the patients is very important to analyse the evolution of breast cancer disease. With these features, our project will permit the users sharing these data. We have created one field *content* to add additional information for each patient but after the meeting with Champalimaud Foundation, we understand that this type of field is not the most appropriate to this area because our web application only allowed sharing text as data and not all important information like the keypoints, bra value, personal information about the patient or even images. These data need to be always up to date so, the app needs to grant to the users the possibility of changing the data whatever they want. Our application permits each user to change the data of each patient and their respective images. Only the patient's owners and user that are members of the same team can update this data. We select three buttons to do these updates:

- Delete - that will delete all the patient data and their respective images.
- Update - that will permit the user updating all the fields about the patient personal information. We create a template with all the fields of the patient and the user can modify all the fields in that template.
- Update Image - will be used to update all the images for each patient or add a new image. Every time that a user wants to update an image we ask for the image ID to be sure that the user is updating the right image. We decided to use the image ID because it is the cleanest an unambiguous way to do this operation. Important to note that when we change an image there is no way to come back and recover the old image. In the same template of Update Image, we have a button to add a new image without deleting others images and we add the possibility of changing the updated data associated with each image. We extract some information about the images but sometimes by many reasons these images are stored without any information to extract and the user may update some metadata values that may be relevant. For instance, the date of the image is one of these values, which is very important to understand the time difference between the date that this image was taken and the date of the surgery. This is of utmost importance for the evaluation of the BCCT method. This difference will be converted in days and will be shown for each image in the patient detail template that we will explain next.

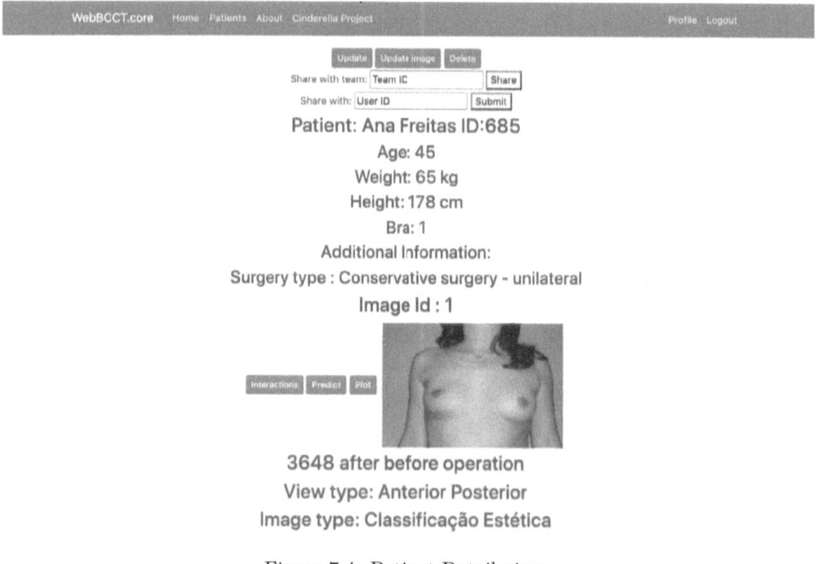

Figure 7.4: Patient Detail view.

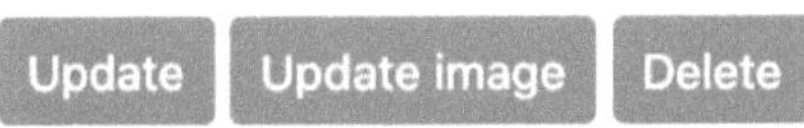

Figure 7.5: Three main buttons of Patient detail.

This template is one of the most informative templates in our project. Here, we show all the information associated with each patient. We created a template with the list of patients for each user. When the user clicks on the patient that he wants to access, a new template will be open and will show all patient information. This is the data which is shown in Figure 7.4. We decided to split the template into two main areas. The first one shows important information like the patient name, age, weight, height, bra and surgery type and the second one shows the information about the images. All this data was discussed in the meeting with the Champalimaud Foundation clinical team, to guarantee that we are implementing the required use-cases. Each image will have some options that the user will be able to complete, like the view type and image type. These data will be shown in the patient template. After the user completes this information, we added the feature mentioned before, the time difference in days, between the surgery date and the date that this photo was taken. For each image, we added the three buttons shown in the Figure 7.5.

- Interactions - This button is used to store and save all the interactions that a user can execute with each patient. It is a very useful tool for our project that permits to see all the important actions that were done for the users and specify who was the author of each interaction and the respective patient. We save the date of each interaction to be easier for users to analyse all the history register. Important to note that these tools were discussed in detail on all the meetings that we had with the specialists in order to create a web application based on the opinions of people who are connected to this area. This button will be used in the future to save interactions made for users with key-functions of our project.
- Predict - This button will run our deep learning model with the respective image by sending the ID of each image and after this model execution is complete we save all the 74 predicted breast keypoint coordinates in our database.
- Plot - This button will draw all the points around the breasts and we will obtain a new template like in 7.6.

These following buttons are in the template generated by the "Plot" button (see Figure 7.6) and are explaining as follow:

- Return to Initial Zoom State - This button resets the current zoom state to the initial zoom state.
- Zoom in and Zoom out - The button "zoom in" will enlarge the image and "zoom-out" shrink the image.

- Update Bra - The button "Update Bra" will save the Bra value in our database.

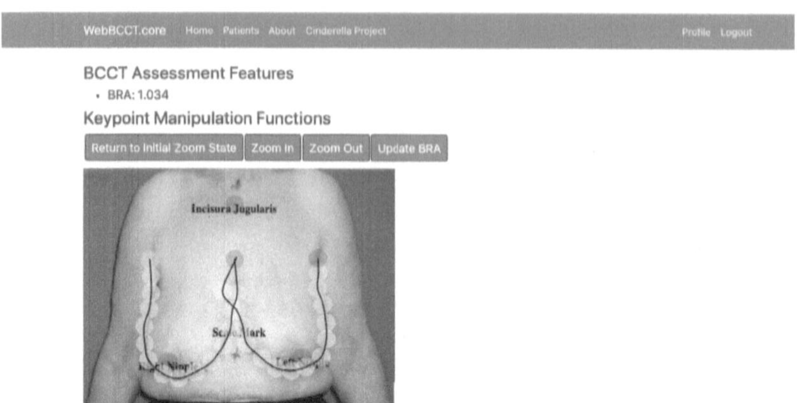

Figure 7.6: Plot, Keypoint Manipulation, Feature Extraction and BCCT classification template.

Chapter 8

Conclusions and Future Work

This chapter summarises the work done in this project and discusses possible suggestions for future work.

8.1 Conclusion

8.1.1 Overview

With this book project, a fully functional back-end of a web application for the aesthetic assessment of breast cancer conservative treatment was designed and implemented.

1. The first phase of this project was focused on the requirements gathering and the definition of milestones. After the decision on the main objectives we planned our tasks to achieve all the goals. First of all, we studied the best tools to use with our project and what were the ones that would bring more advantages to continue the work did before by Gonçalves et al.

2. The second phase was the selection of proper technologies and tools for the implementation of the use-cases and the requirements. After these study cases, we started to develop our project in an iterative way, through weekly tasks. We learned new techniques and the best approaches to develop a web application capable of integrating deep learning models. In this case, is to automatically perform the cosmetic assessment of Breast Cancer Conservative Treatment (BCCT) mentioned before (see Chapter 1).

3. During the third phase, we studied the performance of the web applications and performed quality tests By modifying the entire software architecture and using appropriate tools we developed a successful and efficient web application that permits the execution and integration of deep learning models developed by the group (see Chapter 6).

8.2 Main Contributions

In this project book, we made a brief study of some important technologies used in the development and deployment web. We moved the Breast Cancer Conservative Treatment Cosmetic Results (BCCT.core) to a successful web application, adding new features, capable of integrating deep learning models that will help and improve the quality of the BCCT. With this work, we will help all the people who are involved in the treatment of breast cancer and future developers that aim to produce a web application capable of integrating deep learning algorithms with good performance. There is still space for further improvements, presented in the next section.

8.3 Future Work

8.3.1 Technologies to Improve the User Interface

Every interface and workflow used in our project was discussed and implemented based on the requirements gathering (see Chapter 4). Regarding the current workflow, we consider that will be important to improve the layout to make a more beautiful and user-friendly application. We consider that a study in more detail in technologies like Bootstrap [1]; Backbone.js[2]; React[3] ; AngularJS[4] may be a good approach to start improving our application layout in the future.

8.3.2 Feedback Review

To analyse and ask for an evaluation from the users or even to report some errors about our project we think that this feature will be very important to improve the quality of our service. This feature is very important in all projects to rectify some errors that can appear and to solve some doubts that a user can have. This way we can easily solve the problems of the users and get feedback about some aspects that we should improve.

8.3.3 Private Chat

Nowadays the communication is getting every day faster and some features of sharing knowledge developed by us to share information about patient data, (see Chapter 5), will have a great improvement if we add to these features a chat where it would be possible to all the users talk and comment instantly about some treatment linked with each patient.

8.3.4 Upload Multiple Data

A user-friendly interface which is capable of uploading multiple patient data to each user at the same time.

8.3.5 A Tutorial

One feature that can help the users to work with our application easily is the creation of a tutorial when they make their first login. This feature would help to clarify to the users the usability and will be faster for them to understand the entire work-flow of our project.

8.3.6 Search Engine

After the third and last meeting with the Champalimaud, we understand that is important to create a search engine capable of search for all the attributes regarding with each patient. This would enable users to find some important data linked with investigation purpose.

Appendices

Appendix 1

Entrevista com o Dr. Carlos Mavioso (27-11-2019)

João Rodrigues: *Olá. Eu vou partilhar consigo tudo o que eu tenho para mostrar o documento que abri aqui no meu computador.*

Dr. Carlos Mavioso: *O Tiago tinha mandado isto, mas pode ser assim, pode não ser igual. Aquele onde está até se calhar vejo melhor aqui do que no ecrã do computador, mas vamos lá.*

João Rodrigues: *A minha primeira pergunta é relativamente ao login e à senha. A minha questão é saber qual é, na questão na ótica do utilizador, a forma mais prática de localizar o botão de login e do registo? No documento adicionei algumas opções; se você tiver outra opinião pode dizer. A minha primeira opção é no canto superior direito.*

Dr. Carlos Mavioso: *Sim, eu acho que é intuitiva. Se pensar no caso dos sites dos bancos é quase tudo no canto superior direito. Isso é um bocadinho intuitivo.*

João Rodrigues: *A minha outra pergunta é se pode estar logo implícito no ecrã? Para ser a primeira página a aparecer ao utilizador.*

Dr. Carlos Mavioso: *Sim, o que eu acho é que aparecer logo essa página é fácil de ver ou então no canto superior direito porque é o mais intuitivo. Mas esta hipótese b) também não me parece má porque aparece logo tudo.*

João Rodrigues: *Era por uma questão de ser mais prático.*

Dr. Carlos Mavioso: *Talvez seja mais prático a hipótese b) sim, mas a hipótese a) também é intuitiva.*

João Rodrigues: *Na segunda pergunta que eu faço também relativamente ao login e ao registo, existe aqui um exemplo. Quero dizer, muitas vezes nós queremos fazer login, acha que é prático e é útil para o utilizador ter algum tipo de conta tipo de conta Google, Facebook ou Twitter que seja para o utilizador uma forma mais fácil e simples fazer para login? Não sei até que ponto assinar contas do tipo Google Facebook ou Twitter é mais intuitivo ou não?*

Dr. Carlos Mavioso: *Eu não sei se é muito intuitivo, eu acho que o login como está no quadro anterior deve ser suficiente.*

João Rodrigues: *Só com um username e uma password?*

Dr. Carlos Mavioso: *Acho que sim... pois é assim, não lhe sei não sei dizer muito bem porque eu habitual habitualmente aquilo que vejo nas contas é aquele o quadro de entrada inicial, não me lembro que seja uma utilidade muito grande ter aqui a conta Google, mas acho que isso é até uma questão mais para ver se calhar no futuro. Eu por exemplo não tenho Facebook, portanto, pelo Facebook nunca iria usar porque gente que não tem Facebook e é por isso que não sei se isto poderia ser uma opção... talvez, mas uma opção que não substitua a anterior. Percebo que a pessoa que tem esta conta vai por esta conta, mas eu pessoalmente, para mim, não vejo vantagem.*

João Rodrigues: *A aplicação vai permitir inserir imagens e a minha pergunta é: Qual é a forma mais prática e mais útil de apresentar estes dois botões de inserir ou selecionar a imagem, prefere uma ordem vertical ou horizontal?*

Dr. Carlos Mavioso: *Eu prefiro horizontal, porque a vertical induz um bocadinho em erro no Inserir Imagem. Na horizontal a pessoa olha e tem duas coisas que estão lado a lado e é mais fácil perceber que opção tem, acho que está bem.*

João Rodrigues: *Outra opção que vamos ter é relativa à disposição das imagens, ou seja, podemos apresentá-las com uma lista? Podemos apresentar também como uma grelha...*

Dr. Carlos Mavioso: *Uma coisa, uma dúvida João, aqui nesta primeira na alínea a) em lista, aqui a visualização é só com estes ícones pequenos ou com um ícone a pessoa pode aumentar os ícones? E nesta listagem é um ficheiro com as fotografias e a data das fotografias ou é só um ficheiro?*

João Rodrigues: *Do lado esquerdo temos acesso à lista com o nome das imagens, isto é, o nome das imagens do lado direito.*

Dr. Carlos Mavioso: *As fotografias associadas a cada um destes ficheiros pode puxar um bocadinho para cima a alínea b), eu parece-me que esta é mais fácil... a grelha parece que é mais fácil tem menos informação para nós escolhermos a fotografia, não é?* Visualizando *fotografia, não tem aquela informação toda que está ali eu acho que para quem está a usar se calhar não lhe interessa muito saber qual é o tamanho do GP. Eu pessoalmente gosto mais da alínea b) da grelha.*

João Rodrigues: *Relativamente à manipulação das imagens guardadas na base de dados, vamos ter uma opção que é fazer o zoom-in na imagem, manipular a imagem; e uma das minhas dúvidas é saber onde posso adicionar o botão e qual é a, perante a imagem, o sítio mais prático para adicionar o botão? Eu adicionei aqui no canto superior direito.*

Dr. Carlos Mavioso: *Sim, no meio da fotografia não me parece lógico, eu acho que ou no canto superior direito ou no canto superior esquerdo, mas a tendência é que a pessoa vá sempre ao canto superior direito porque é onde normalmente estão as opções nas outras coisas. Acho que o superior direito ficaria bem relativamente à localização do botão.*

João Rodrigues: *Relativamente ao botão de "upload Image", era se inserir no meio do ecrã, no topo do ecrã ou um sistema "drag and drop"? Em que tem a imagem onde seleciona e arrasta somente para o site e o site carrega.*

Dr. Carlos Mavioso: *O drag and drop é fácil mas eu acho que a alínea a), quando carregamos aqui no "upload Image" aí no meio depois aparece uma coisa para selecionar o ficheiro? Certo?*

João Rodrigues: *Certo.*

Dr. Carlos Mavioso: *Eu ou esta ou a outra do arrastar, ou uma ou outra. Talvez a outra escolha do ficheiro seja mais fácil porque é o que habitualmente se faz mais, mas o drag and drop não é uma coisa que eu acho que seja difícil de fazer.*

João Rodrigues: *Relativamente ao feedback. Há várias formas de o fazer, na ótica do utilizador é sempre um bocado chato fazer o feedback porque está sempre a perder tempo e eu queria perguntar qual era a forma menos dolorosa para o utilizador dar o feedback. Eu diria que há várias opções. A primeira é enviar um e-mail com um link onde segue o questionário a pessoa responde ao questionário ou fazer um questionário com várias métricas de avaliação, ou seja, ter uma pergunta e a forma de responder varia ou deveria ter um questionário com respostas diretas à pergunta, isto é, a resposta está implícita? E uma simples escala onde a resposta é direta.*

Dr. Carlos Mavioso: *Eu acho o seguinte a maior parte das pessoas quer dar um feedback que seja o mais rápido possível e o menos, entre aspas, chato. Das duas uma: ou a pessoa tem um questionário, mas um questionário simples, muito pequeno em que as respostas são de escolha múltipla e resolve-se rapidamente o questionário. Porque estar a escrever a maior parte das pessoas não vai aderir; ou então esta ideia do fim em que tem só uma escala com estrelas de uma a cinco estrelas, dando sempre a hipótese ao utilizador para enviar um email para justificar aquilo que acha que correu melhor ou pior dentro da sua impressão da aplicação. Mas se fizerem um questionário simples também não acho mal, acho que tem que se escolher muito bem as perguntas que se vão fazer e a forma de responder ser direta, tipo escala. Uma coisa desse género. A opção d) é a mais fácil, mas também se calhar é aquela onde o João vai ter menos informação acerca uma opinião mais correta sobre as coisas. Se houver um questionário como, pode puxar um bocadinho para cima...*

João Rodrigues: *Sim, sim.*

Dr. Carlos Mavioso: *O b) por exemplo, com perguntas muito simples e com uma escala para responder sim ou não, ou então classificar de 1 a 5. Mas também não pôr muitas perguntas, porque muitas mais que três, mais que três ou quatro perguntas se calhar é um bocadinho demais e da mesma forma deixar em aberto a hipótese de haver um feedback via email. Percebe? Eu acho que seria uma boa hipótese.*

João Rodrigues: *Relativamente à estrutura de dados. A nossa ideia é ter um user que pode ter vários projetos em cada projeto está inserido a localização do projeto, um projeto_id, que vai identificar o projeto e cada projeto tem associado as suas fotos. Uma das minhas questões tendo em conta estas entidades que estão aqui na base na base de dados é se acha útil ou acha necessário adicionar mais entidades à relação, do género: ao user, na altura, adicionei o user_id, o nome, o email, o nome do usuário, foto do user.*

Dr. Carlos Mavioso: *Eu acho que a foto do user não deve ser uma opção obrigatória, deve ser uma opção, não deve ser uma coisa obrigatória porque muita gente não gosta de partilhar a foto. E eu acho que pode pôr a foto, mas opcional, enquanto as outras coisas têm que ser. Tem que ser uma coisa que a pessoa tem de preencher porque a gente precisa de saber quem está a usar e com que frequência e como está a usar, a fotografia eu acho que se calhar é pedir um bocadinho mais ao utilizador.*

João Rodrigues: *Ok. Uma das minhas perguntas também é saber se acha prático e útil para um utilizador ter acesso a vários projetos ou se um utilizador ter acesso só aos seus projetos ou só a um único projeto?*

Dr. Carlos Mavioso: *Eu acho que ele pode ter acesso a mais que um projeto, não é? Claro, que participando nesse projeto, não é? Porque não sei até que ponto deve ter acesso a projetos nos quais ele não participa. Acho que sim.*

João Rodrigues: *Uma das questões que me ocorreu, foi saber se acha que é importante ter um admin do projeto?*

Dr. Carlos Mavioso: *Não lhe sei dizer.*

João Rodrigues: *Acha que era útil ter um limite ou não de fotos? Ou seja, Todos os utilizadores podem adicionar todas as fotos que queiram ou ter um número limitado de fotos.*

Dr. Carlos Mavioso: *Pelo que eu percebi o objetivo de fazer esta base de dados é ter o máximo possível de fotos de aprendizagem. Acho que não deveria haver um limite de fotos, pode ser que haja alguma limitação na base de dados ou uma coisa assim não sei.*

João Rodrigues: *Ok, acho que da base de dados está tudo. Qual é para si o melhor método de exportação dos dados guardados na base de dados? E qual era o tipo de ficheiro mais fácil para exportação e para manipulação dos dados?*

Dr. Carlos Mavioso: *XLSX, os outros não me dizem absolutamente nada.*

Tiago Gonçalves: *Acho que da minha parte minha parte eu só quero fazer uma intervenção. Nós podemos ter um projeto com fotos de vários pacientes e seria um projeto diferente, ou se a cada projeto, por exemplo, seria associado um só paciente com diversas fotos desse mesmo paciente, e nós queremos ver como é que é feita essa organização. Se é feita, vamos supor, por projeto, ou por caso de estudo com determinadas datas, se é por o paciente; como é que acha que seria mais útil? A ideia dos projetos surge nesta onde onda.*

Dr. Carlos Mavioso: *Por paciente fica mais fácil distinguir a sequência de fotos que supõe certo? Imagine eu tenho o paciente A B C e D e a determinada altura eu quero carregar uma fotografia do paciente A num determinado tempo, que é um pós-operatório e que eu quero avaliar, certo? Pronto. Imagine que esse doente e também o B e o C para fazer o mesmo tipo de avaliação. Mas imagine que o paciente A mais tarde volta a fazer uma nova uma nova cirurgia para melhorar um aspeto, qualquer coisa, e eu vou inseri-lo novamente. Talvez tenha que haver uma forma de nós percebermos que é o mesmo doente numa sequência diferente, numa fase diferente.*

Tiago Gonçalves: *Ok. Se calhar, o que sugere é termos um projeto e esse projeto, eu estou a chamar projeto, mas pode ter outro nome, por exemplo relativo a um só paciente e depois dentro desse projeto agrupar as fotos desse paciente numa linha temporal seria mais interessante?*

Dr. Carlos Mavioso: *Não quer dizer que todos os doentes vão ter várias cirurgias e várias fotografias pós-operatórios, a maioria deles provavelmente vai ter só uma. Mas temos que se calhar temos que deixar em aberto a hipótese de pôr mais que uma fotografia por doente num espaço temporal diferente, até porque às vezes nós podemos querer avaliar mesmo não tendo havido uma nova cirurgia, queremos avaliar uma evolução no tempo. Imagine, tiramos uma fotografia hoje e daqui a um ano voltamos a tirar. Queremos ver como é que o software avalia a evolução. Como é que ficou. Se calhar poderíamos ter essa hipótese dentro de cada doente. Poder pôr mais que uma foto para percebermos que é o mesmo doente. Porque se o objetivo último é o software aprender alguma coisa também temos que dar como hipótese, a de ele perceber que aquilo é a mesma coisa numa fase diferente.*

Tiago Gonçalves: *Sim, sim, haver uma organização e assim não confundir de certa forma a aprendizagem do software.*

Dr. Carlos Mavioso: *Se nós não fizermos isso, se o utilizador colocar a fotografia de um doente que já pôs antes e não informar que aquela fotografia já foi posta; e se calhar é uma coisa que nós temos que ter explicito para aos utilizadores e que cada doente que é colocado depois se voltar a colocar fotografia se calhar tem que alocar aquela, que é aquele corpo como vocës chamam, o projeto, o projeto daquele doente porque senão estamos a pôr fotografias do mesmo doente em tempos diferentes que não sei, até que ponto isso ajuda; talvez ajude mais sabendo que é aquele mesmo doente num tempo diferente.*

Tiago Gonçalves: *Se esse nome, esse projeto então poderia chamar-se paciente e, entretanto, seríamos, de certa forma, ligar diferentes clínicos a esse mesmo paciente havendo aquela partilha que o João falou há bocado, ou seja, de diferentes pessoas a estudar aquela que é o caso do caso clínico.*

Dr. Carlos Mavioso: *Por exemplo.*

Tiago Gonçalves: *Ok, essa era uma pergunta. Por acaso, tinha-me surgido que não sabíamos muito bem como é que era feita a organização, mas acho que sua resposta já nos deu uma luz sobre aquilo que temos que fazer e acho que sim, porque no limite podemos ter uma opção em que por exemplo vamos supor que o utilizador quer utilizar o software para uma outra coisa, vamos dar um exemplo, fins pedagógicos, e o programa consegue ir buscar fotografias diferentes. Aí torna-as anónimas, por exemplo, a alguns alunos e não mostra o paciente. Uma última pergunta, por acaso a nossa reunião está a ser bastante direta, é uma coisa boa. Outra pergunta era se se o Doutor se lembra de alguma função que nós não tínhamos abordado e que achasse pertinente que um software deste género, baseado na sua experiência, que é que se tivesse que escolher uma coisa que nunca viu ser feita ou implementada, se se lembrar, o que seria interessante para você?*

Dr. Carlos Mavioso: *Tiago, o software que a gente vai usar é o BCCT.core, não é? Que eu já usei para fazer aquelas fotografias, não é? Eu acho bastante intuitivo, bastante fácil de usar assim. Se me lembrar até digo, que eu adorei fazer aquilo, e fiz algumas 500 ou 600 fotografias numa penada só porque acho que é muito fácil e não estou a ver nada que se possa acrescentar porque eu acho que está bom, é muito fácil de utilizar e é isso que importa mas se me lembrar de alguma coisa certamente entro em contacto convosco.*

Tiago Gonçalves: *Certíssimo, esta pergunta vem mesmo nesse sentido pronto, é uma necessidade que cada vez mais, pelo menos da parte de engenharia e também da parte clínica, há a necessidade de fazer coisas que as pessoas usem e gostem de usar, esta pergunta surge no caso de se lembrar de alguma coisa.*

Dr. Carlos Mavioso: *É muito fácil de usar e eu acho que se calhar pôr mais qualquer coisa até vai prejudicar.*

Tiago Gonçalves: *Certíssimo, certíssimo. Uma outra opção que nós temos é que do ponto de vista da engenharia e acredito que será para os clínicos também possa ser é, ou seja, os nossos algoritmos adaptam-se consoante os dados que vamos fornecendo, ou seja, vão aprender. Eu não sei, se acha interessante, por exemplo, um determinado clínico ter um paciente ou um determinado grupo de pacientes e que tentasse fazer com que o algoritmo funcionasse bem naquele determinado grupo de pacientes? Forçando o software de certa forma a treinar. Seria interessante isto acontecer, ou seja, de forma visível para o clínico? Acharia interessante que este treino do algoritmo da inteligência por trás fosse feita de forma mais discreta sem prejudicar a usabilidade por parte do clínico?*

Dr. Carlos Mavioso: *Eu acho que a segunda hipótese é talvez melhor.*

Tiago Gonçalves: *Pronto. Eu não tenho atualmente mais nenhuma pergunta. O Professor Jaime atrasou-se mais um bocado que ele teve um compromisso, por isso é que ele não pôde estar cá. Não sei se tem alguma dúvida que queira colocar?*

Dr. Carlos Mavioso: *Para já não tenho nenhuma dúvida se depois houver alguma coisa eu ligo ao Jaime ou alguma coisa assim.*

João Rodrigues: *Em relação à proteção de dados até que ponto agora posso guardar diretamente na minha base de dados o nome do "user"?*

Dr. Carlos Mavioso: *Isso não lhe sei responder. Mas eu acho que cabe à partida perguntar ao utilizador se vai autorizar ser identificado ou não quando estão a aceder à base de dados dessa pessoa.*

João Rodrigues: *Ok, ok.*

Tiago Gonçalves: *Pronto. Doutor Carlos, uma vez mais quero lhe agradecer o seu tempo. Entretanto vamos descarregar o vídeo de gravação da chamada e vamos transcrever. Já será o trabalho do João e depois iremos reenviar para termos a aprovação de que aquilo está no documento, se falou aqui. E assim é uma fonte de informação que o João já poderá integrar na tese ou utilizar para fazer a tese e assim ajudará mais. Eu agradecia-lhe, uma vez mais, o seu tempo. Da nossa parte acho que é tudo, obrigado.*

João Rodrigues: *Obrigado Tiago, Dr. Carlos, mais uma vez, pela atenção.*

Dr. Carlos Mavioso: *Qualquer coisa, liguem está bem?*

Tiago Gonçalves: *Ok. Muito obrigado, continuação de um bom trabalho.*

www.ingramcontent.com/pod-product-compliance
Lightning Source LLC
LaVergne TN
LVHW090134160826
845673LV00017B/2462
9783384242501